A new view of real cause and real cure for diseases

The simple exercises help to warm the hands, self-reduce the pain and headache in just 10 minutes.

Natural techniques that can help to treat:

- Asthma
- Bronchitis
- Cold
- COPD
- Coughing
- Difficult breathing
- Fever
- Flu A

- Alzheimer's diseases
- Backache
- Dizziness
- Eye problems
- Headache
- Insomnia
- Nerve pain
- Parkinson

- Cancer
- Diabetes
- Fatigue
- Fibromyalgia
- Hypertension
- Hypotension
- Hemorrhoid
- Gastritis

We will discuss in this book how to self-removing the trigger point and balancing metabolic reactions

The keys to fatigue, backache, headache, leg pain, neurodegenerative diseases, asthma, COPD, flu, fever, flu A, and COVID-19.

As a pharmacist and I have using these techniques to help hundreds of patients with these simple techniques, I just want to describe these in the view of science and modern medicine.

Let's do the self-diagnosing to see if you have it.

Self-checking the health and finding the trigger points
Just press the thumb on the stomach of people: right upper stomach (liver), Left upper stomach (gastric), and middle-lower stomach (intestine, ovule or prostate), if it pain, there may be block for fluidity
Quick and slight clap on the shoulder, neck, back, lumbar, head, and forehead to see if there are the sensations of pain, piercing, burning, or comfortable.
Check the hands, feet to feel if it warm, and scratch on the feet to feel if there are abnormal feelings
Bend and the neck and the back to see if it feels uncomfortable. Turning the head to the left and to the right to see if it have uncomfortable
Pressing along the eyebrows to see if there is pain or piercing.
Clapping or quick punching on the chest to see if it is pain, piercing or comfortable feelings.

The stomach, a place where digestion, absorption, and elimination has taken place, should be in a good state.

- In Vietnam, we are told to put a small blanket across the stomach of the kids during the sleep to make them sleep well and not ill.

- In traditional, when people have cold stomach pain, we are told to rub the topical hot medical ointments, drink sweet ginger juice or massage the stomach.

These facts and the experience make I think of the vital role of blood circulation in health and chronic illness. Poor blood circulation may come from the blocking points in the vessels or from low blood pressure or low blood glucose. In the body, all the billions of cells of all body systems need the energy to have normal functions; which is mainly generated from metabolizing glucose. When the cells hunger for glucose, it can start to use structure stored glucose or stored lipids or polysaccharides or structure lipid or structure protein. To take stored glucose, the body needs good blood circulation and right body temperature. The people with chronic illness often have hormonal imbalanced – which need glucose as the main source of energy also, and poor blood circulation and disorder of thermoregulation. If we do not stop these disorders, these people may have metabolic disorders or metabolic diseases. The main energy source for the cells is from the catabolism of glucose. So any problem for glycemia and oxygen saturation will make the billions of cells of the body are out of balance.

A metabolic disorder can generate free oxygen and free radicals. On the other hand, the immune system is not in a good state because of the hunger for energy may fail in repairing the damage caused by metabolic disorders.

In traditional medicine, the pain mainly caused by trigger points, so all alternative therapies like acupressure, dry needle, massage aim to remove trigger points. In the metabolic view, I saw that the trigger points mainly in the muscle which presses the surrounding vessels of blood circulation. The signs of trigger point are pain, numbness, coldness, or rigidness. Poor blood circulation may make the target cells and target organs hunger for the glucose and poison by the metabolic wastes which are not carried out well by the poor blood circulation.

Glycemia, oxygen saturation and blood pressure are mainly control by heart, vessels, liver, pancreatic, intestine, lungs and kidneys. Any problems that happen to the heart, vessels, liver, pancreatic, intestine, lungs or kidneys will make the whole body have the various problems described by syndromes or metabolic diseases. Only oxygen can not create energy, the body does not have stored oxygen we do need breath continuously. To have a good metabolism, the blood needs to supply glucose or substrates for the cells at the optimum levels. Supplying substrate for metabolic reactions depend on the blood circulation to carried stored glucose and stored lipid in the abdominal area.

We can only heal the chronic illness in a short time when we understand:

"ALL IN ONE,

AND ONE REPRESENTS ALL"

This book is dedicated to

My mother, Muot T. Nguyen, my fathers: Dung D. Dao and Thinh N. Duc, my wife, Hoa N. T. Kieu, and my children: Khang, Khai, whom I learn the most and motivate me the most to write the book.

I want to say thank all Is, speakers, teachers who give me invaluable materials, proofs, citations, references, and instructions to write this book directly and indirectly. I really appreciate and want to say thank them all. I thank the authors listed on the references in this book. Their works, teachings, and findings have shaped my mind.

I also want to say thank all my teachers, friends, colleagues, brothers, and sisters because of their work, their supports have shaped my mind.

I want to thank the Vietnamese government has to support invaluable chances for me to work, study, and access to advanced knowledge with an incredible price.

Best of all, I want to thank you :___(Your name)__

You are the readers chose to participate with me on the way to help the needed people. You are my greatest inspiration for me to finish the work. And I know that together we can help more. You are approved for fair use of any part which less than 1000 words.

My webs my help:

Awakenyouwonderfulwe.com

Daoduyvan.com

Hanoi, 26/09/2017

Van Duy Dao

Chapter I: New view of self healing.

1. In practice as a pharmacist, I found new view of pain, diseases and self healing.

In practice, the saw that when glycemia below the normal level, most practitioners feel dizziness, vertigo, weakness, these signs can be deal well with just a glass of sugar juice. This makes I realized that glycemia, blood pressure, and physical health is interdependent. People have good health when they have these indicators in the normal range. It is also the aim that most traditional aim to deal with. The traditional medicine aims to solve the cause and make the whole body is balanced. Modern medicine merely treats the symptoms which are the results metabolism disordered.

When we talk about the vital role of oxygen, we forget that the vital role of oxygen is to interact with glucose in the cells catalyzed by many enzymes to generate energy. The main source to generate energy in cells is from glucose, enough glucose is as vital as enough oxygen. Poor blood circulation may come from the blocking points in the vessels or from low blood pressure or low blood glucose. In the body, all the billions of cells of all body systems need the energy to have normal functions; which is mainly generated from metabolizing glucose. When the cells hunger for glucose, it can start to use structure stored glucose or stored lipids or polysaccharides or structure lipid or structure protein. To take stored glucose, the body needs good blood circulation and right body temperature. The people with chronic illness often have hormonal imbalanced – which need glucose as the main source of energy also, and poor blood circulation and disorder of thermoregulation. If we do not stop these disorders, these people may have metabolic disorders or metabolic diseases. The main energy source for the cells is from the catabolism of

1

glucose. So any problem for glycemia and oxygen saturation will make the billions of cells of the body are out of balance. During practice Vietnamese Qi gong combining with traditional medicine, I realized that in just ten minutes, just by removing trigger point and balancing metabolic reactions, we can deal easily most of the symptoms of fatigue, nerve pain, chronic illness, diabetes, fibromyalgia, Alzheimer's diseases, Vestibular disorder, and Neurodegenerative Diseases.

Smokers inhale nicotine and many other chemicals in the cigarettes which increase the metabolism in the body because of smoking speeds up the metabolism, so the body burns calories at a faster rate. When people stop smoking, they actually need fewer calories so they will put on weight when they quit. But why do not smokers have the feeling of hunger compared to when they quit smoking? When they smoke, they do inhale nicotine, which leads to consuming a lot of energy so they should have the feeling of hunger more than when they quit smoking. But in fact, the smokers do not have the feeling of hunger. This leads to the paradox of smoking that is unanswered: "consume more energy but feeling less hungry. Quitting smoke, in metabolism, will make the body consumes less energy, but why do they have more the feeling of hunger than when they smoke. Some scientists explained that smoking can suppress the appetite of the smoker to answer why quitting smoke will make more feeling of hunger for food; this explanation is wrong because many smokers still have a good appetite. Teachings the breathing in Qi Gong, I found that it is in the mechanism of deep breathing via the mouth can increase the mobilizing glucose from the body into the bloodstream. We do know that the level of glucose in the body has a relation to the feeling of hunger. This review will show the forgotten clues to explain this paradox. The answer may be in a deep breath by mouth which leads to mobilizing all organs in the

2

stomach unintentionally. The rhythmic moving of the billions of cells and organs in the stomach may increase the blood flow in the intestine, the stomach, the liver, the kidney, the oval, and many other important organs which make the metabolism of the stomach increased substantially. The answer is the unintentional diaphragm breath make the circulation and metabolism of the stomach increased substantially; which need more research to find real application in medical practice.

Table 1: Self-checking the health and trigger points before, during and after practicing self-healing techniques or any other treatment.

Self-checking the health and trigger points	
It is not good if it is higher or lower than normal. It indicates that there are some forgotten health problems.	Checking the blood pressure on both hands several times a day to see if it is normal, low or high
	Checking glycemia when you hungry, tired, and after eating, drinking sweet juice to see if it is normal.
Check the state of the important organs in the stomach.	Just press the thumb on the stomach of people: right upper stomach (liver), Left upper stomach (gastric), and middle-lower stomach (intestine, ovule or prostate), if it pain, there may be block for fluidity
Forgotten trigger points along the way will make people have abnormal sensations.	Quick and slight clap on the shoulder, neck, back, lumbar, head, and forehead to see if there are the sensations of pain, piercing, burning, or comfortable.

Checking blood circulation to the feet, hands	Check the hands, feet to feel if it warm, and scratch on the feet to feel if there are abnormal feelings
Check the blood circulation to the head well or not	Bend and the neck and the back to see if it feels uncomfortable. Close the eyes than sit down and stand up 10 times to see you have the feeling of dizziness or vertigo. Turning the head to the left and to the right to see if it have uncomfortable
Check the blood circulation to the eyes	Pressing along the eyebrows to see if there is pain or piercing.
Check the health of the lungs	Clapping or quick punching on the chest to see if it is pain, piercing or comfortable feelings.
Self-finding any trigger points on the body	Clapping and pressing many points in the body to see if there are abnormal feelings.

Applying Vietnamese Qi Gong instructed by master Do Duc Ngoc, and other simple physical exercises to help treating the chronic diseases.

Table 2: Self-healing techniques and physical therapies that boost blood circulation,

Self-healing exercises that boost blood circulation	
	Benefits
Clapping create rhythmic impacts on the organs in the hollow	

covered by bones and muscles.

Rhythmic pressing used to have impacts on the organs in the soft parts of the body like the abdominals

Eat and drink first to equip the body enough energy for self-healing	Equipt blood with enough nutrition and normal glycemia.
Tie the calf by an elastic crepe or an elastic rubber band then walks on a step or stair for 10 minutes. Just tie it comfortably, not too strick to prevent blood circulation.	Walking with comfortable tying the calves creates a rhythmic strong impact on the arteries in the legs and blood circulation when we walk the step.
Lie down and place an object on the lower abdomen: the place between the navel and genital organs.	Pressing rhythmic forces by the rhythm of breathing. Rhythmic forces will have impacts on blood circulation and the organs in the stomach like cervical, large intestine, kidneys, liver, small intestine, prostate. By placing an object, relax, closing the eyes, the object will catch the attention of the conscious mind that will make the mind empty and relaxed which creates good sleep and reduce stress.
Relaxed deep breathing, by pronouncing the long and small sound when breathing out, we can have deep breathing naturally	Lots of benefit from deep breathing recognized by the traditional therapist, modern doctors and Qigong masters It also, help to mobilized all organs in the abdominal naturally with the rhythm of

	relaxed breathing.
Clapping on trigger points until having the sensation of roughness. Clap on the muscle of the back, the shoulder, the neck, the nape, and the head when the body and hands are warm	All the points of acupuncture, acupressure, traditional therapies, and massage therapies aim at will have rhythmic impact by suitable clapping. Clap till have the feeling of roughness, we do know that the impacts of this clapping just make normal skins feel roughness (test on the normal skins of the body), it means that the trigger points have been removed.
Finding and removing trigger points in the lungs by quickly clapping or punching on chest and the upper back	Just try quick clapping on the table, we will see the objects on the table vibrates, so when we do this on chest and back, all vessels and tissues will vibrate. This will help to clear the cloths, dust and trigger points in the lungs and bronchi
Removing trigger points in the organs in the abdominal by pulling the knee to the chest and blow the air deeply and slowly. Breathe in and out via mouth. We can put the towel on the abdominal to have more forces on the organs.	Boost the blood circulation on the whole body and on the target organ in the stomach like liver, gastric, intestine, pancreas, prostate, kidneys, ovules…
Loading energy, boosting blood circulation for five important organsPlaces 2 plates	Stand like this for 5 to 10 minutes to make the body and the back warm or sweating. In

together on the floor. Stand with your feet slightly broader than shoulder-width, then twist the feet to make the toes move closer together, the toes make a V shape. Then bend the knees to make the 2 knees against each other, lower the body part, still keep the back upright, Stretch the arms in front keeping the fingers together then the palms up.	twisting the feet, all muscles are much stretcher than not twisting the feet. This boost the blood circulation very well, stretching all the muscles very much so that the body will have sweating in just 5 or 10 minutes.
Losen all the muscle of the hands, flap or swing the hands and fast as possible, for 10 minutes	We can clap on the back of other people, or on the table, chair, in the air or on trees. When loosening the muscle and flapping the hands, the blood will circulate well, the muscle will be softened, and well fed. Do this can make the body warm and have sweating, it has a great impact on making ill people stop fever, reduce the pain and irritation.

Exercise of breathing that practitioners can self do it, it is better to have blood pressure machine and glucose blood checker machine to see the impacts on the body and metabolism inside the body. Always check the warm and the humidity in the palms of the hands.

Physiotherapy can help but too complicated for all.

Back to the root of physical techniques, and traditional medical techniques, and regular physical exercise we can see that by suitable and physical forces, we can create the health outcomes. The techniques may be different but they all aim to boost the blood circulation. Its advantages can help us have health outcomes but it may too complicated for all people to self doing it.

But when we know all the aim of these physical therapies are to boost the blood circulation to the weak or ill organs, untrained people can self do it to have good blood circulation to the target organs. By self-diagnosing, we can know the organs are in good state or ill. And by the suitable exercise in just 10 minutes, we can increase the blood circulation to the target organs which carried oxygen and nutritions and carried out harmful wastes so well that we can feel comfortable immediately.

Physical therapy, also known as physiotherapy, treats acute or chronic pain, movement and physical impairments resulting from injury, trauma or illness typically of musculoskeletal, cardiovascular, respiratory, neurological, and endocrinological origins. Physical therapy is used to improve a patient's physical functions through physical examination, diagnosis, prognosis, patient education, physical intervention, rehabilitation, disease prevention and health promotion.

The health symptoms and diseases can benefit from these exercises:

The common advice for all these health problems are having suitable exercise and having the right diet. Baking soda, papaya, fruits, vitamins, minerals, alternative therapies, and traditional medicine also play an important role in dealing with these diseases. If there are a lot of trigger points or blocking points around the vessels, it will make the distribution of the glucose and oxygen in the body disorder. On the other hand, there are many sensors of the autonomic nervous system that lie along the vessels in the head, liver, legs, hands and all other

8

organs to have the autonomic responses to maintain balanced homeostasis. The chronic trigger points will create longterm changes in the homeostasis and make the autonomic nervous system out of balance. To some extent, traditional therapies, suitable diets, and alternative therapies seem to be effective for treating some chronic diseases because these therapies help to remove trigger points.

• To make the hand warm, reduce irritation in patients who have Raynaud

• Removing backache, pain in the neck and headache.

• Removing Vestibular disorder hay vestibular trouble

• To remove the headache, dizziness, vertigo and floating and most of the symptoms of Alzheimer's and neurodegenerative Diseases

• Preventing Alzheimer's & neurodegenerative Diseases

• Removing numbness and tingling in hands and feet.

• Removing the weakness and hands and legs

• Removing lumbar pain

• Making balancing for diabetes patients

• Reducing blood pressure by removing the trigger points, the resistance of the vessels will back to normal.

• Preventing heart failure, renal failure

• Liver inflammation relating to the poor blood circulation into the liver

• Heart pain relating to the poor blood circulation to the heart

• Intestine problems relating to the poor blood circulation to the intestine systems: irritation bowel movement, chronic diarrhea, chronic constipation

• Removing nerve pain and nerve inflammation

• Removing chronic fatigue.

• Treating insomnia because it increases the blood circulation to the brain and placing a small object on the lower stomach will make people pay attention to it during breathing, which can make their head is empty from unwanted thinking.

• Stress makes the blood circulation and the whole body imbalanced

• Chronic poor blood circulation can make people suffer hypoglycemia, hypotension. These symptoms make be found in localize organs or localized tissue or the whole body.

Natural healing for all acute and chronic diseases from applying suitable exercise that boost blood circulation and the right nutrition

Mechanism of alternative therapies that help to prevent and heal chronic illness aim at nutritions and removing harmful wastes and clearing the vessels

Table 3: Mechanism of alternative therapies that help to prevent and heal chronic illness aim at nutritions and removing harmful wastes and clearing the vessels

Mechanism of most application on preventing and healing chronic illness
To make the metabolic reactions have optimum rate, blood circulation, PH, nature of the substrate, temperature, enzymes, the concentration of substrate, the concentration of products, repairing damages, immune cells, homeostatic, motility of surrounding fluid should be at the optimum levels.
1. Aspirin, papaya, baking soda, acupressure, massage, statin drugs, and NSAIDs help to prevent and remove the blood clots, trigger points in the vessels and tissues.

10

2. Exercise, suitable physical laboring work increases blood circulation, fluid mobility, and exchanging particles between blood and cells.

3. Vitamins, minerals in fruits and balanced diets play an important role in contributing substrates and activating enzymes. Enzymes are important for all metabolic reactions.

4. Vitamines also play important roles as the antioxidants. Herbs help to reduce free oxidants. Sweating help to remove harmful wastes along with the sweat.

5. Mindfulness, meditation, and positive affirmation help the body relaxed and in balanced which facilitates the process of healing and preventing blood clots, free oxidants and free radical. Most of the techniques are deep breath, observe the breath, or relaxed abdominal breathing.

6. Baking soda reduces PH acid from disorder metabolism. PH acid is not good for the cells, tissues, and metabolism. Facilitate the blood circulation can help to make the metabolism in balanced. We do know that the magical healing of the body, just clear the way, we can see it immediately

7. Deep breathing and diaphragm breathing help to mobilize all cells, tissues, and organs of important systems in the abdominal, which increases the temperature of the abdomen, makes the abdomen softer more flexible than before. This breathing also increases the blood circulation between organs, increase rate, and efficiency of the metabolic and catabolic in the abdomens. This leads to increasing the metabolic rate of the whole body.

8. Balanced diets may make all participants of metabolism at an optimum level: macrobiotic, balanced diets, or rich fruits diet. In all normal diets contained glucid, proteins, and lipids. In food, there are little vitamines, minerals.

Top ten causes of death in high income/affluent countries – lazy lifestyle diseases, right understanding is the lazy lifestyle do not help the blood circulation. Right exercise that can help blood circulations can help these diseases.

Table 4: Top ten causes of death in high income/affluent countries – lifestyle diseases

Top ten causes of death in high income/affluent countries
1. Ischemic heart diseases
2. Stroke
3. Alzheimer disease and other dementia
4. Trachea, bronchus and lung cancer
5. Chronic obstructive pulmonary disease
6. Lower respiratory infections
7. Colon and rectum cancers
8. Diabetes
9. Kidney diseases
1. Breast cancer

2. Effect of deep breathing, Vietnamese Qi Gong exercise, and smoking on glycemia.

It is deep breathing, not the smoke, which makes people lose weight. It is the diaphragm breath, not the smoke, to reduce the rate of getting Parkinson's disease. The obvious fact is the deep breathing by the mouth of the smokers can reduce the rate of getting Parkinson's disease.

Respiration therapy in Khi Cong Y Dao Vietnam, an alternative form of health exercise founded by Master Do Duc Ngoc in 1980, Master Do is widely respected by many people for his expert knowledge of the ancient Eastern concept "Qi" or "Chi" energy. At its core, Khi Cong Y Dao Vietnam combines the idea of Chi energy with simple, specific physical exercises, which is able to stimulate the body to repair damage and regenerate itself. The nutrition, herbs, sugar intake, and suitable physical exercises of Vietnamese Qi Gong can make us gain most of the results of most alternative therapies.

Inner exercise: best of all is the exercise for the stomach. We do know the good effect of deep breathing in yoga, Qi gong, and meditation. We do know the negative effect of shallow, quick breathing. During my practice, I discover that this relationship to the metabolism of the billions of cells in the abdomen areas which can be a trigger to increase multifold just by practicing. The deep breathing and normal breathing do not change much in the volume of the lungs, but it is relating to the voluntary movement of the stomach muscle and diaphragm muscle during the deep breathing, this leads to the activation of billons cells of many organs in the stomach accidentally. This process increase the blood flow to the stomach, increase the glycemia to the stomach cells, this makes the semi-rigid cells in the stomach activate again. Just a little of practicing the deep breathing by mouth, practitioners may feel the stomach more soften and warmer than before. This is the signs that the cells activate again, the inactivate cells or semi inactive cells activate fully again. The full activation of the billions of cells in the organs still continue after stop practicing the breath, because I can still see the glycemia of practitioners still reducing when they take the rest, some practitioners still feel tired after practicing so that they have to take glasses of sugar juice to feel well again. The activated cells may uptake the sugar in the blood too much to compensate for the hunger of the cells for too long. It is like the cells may bright up with the practicing of deep breathing like the experiment of the dr Dang Chi Van found in the cancerous cells in mice brighten up when let the mice drink the juice have baking soda. In other words, all the cells in the stomach may have full metabolism as normal cells. Why deep breathing is so effective: firstly, it is synergy with the breath to continuously activate the cells in the abdomen so that practitioners do not feel tired. Secondly, is not the breath, but the activation of the billions of cells in the stomach and increase the blood flow to stomach areas gradually, leading to the metabolism of the billions of cells activated then the functions of repairing the damage and removing the temporary blockages in the vessels and organs are at a peak. Metabolism, blood flow, balanced glycemia, and the heat will make all enzymes in the stomach at peak of actions, these enzymes are vital for repairing, removing, controlling, and active transporting functions of the cells in the stomach. Just by placing an object in the lower abdomen in lying posture, then slowly breath by mouth can make people feel warm in the abdomen, hands, and feet – even the ones who always have cold hand and cold feet.

To make the stomach, a place where digestion, absorption, and elimination has taken place, in a good state

---

In Vietnam, we are told to put a small blanket across the stomach of the kids during sleep to make them sleep well and not ill.

In traditional, when people have cold stomach pain, we are told to rub the topical hot medical ointments, drink sweet

---

ginger juice or massage the stomach

Due to the lung expansion being lower (inferior) on the body as opposed to higher up (superior), it is referred to as 'deep' and the higher lung expansion of the rib cage breathing is referred to as 'shallow'. The actual volume of air taken into the lungs with either means vary.

Several conditions are marked by or are symptomatic of, shallow breathing. The more common of these conditions include   various anxiety disorders, asthma, hyperventilation, pneumonia, pulmonary edema,   and shock. Anxiety, stress,   and panic   attacks often accompany shallow breathing.

Before the test, we check the blood pressure: systolic pressure/diastolic pressure. Then during the breathing, we check the blood pressure regularly, and when the participants said they have some strange feeling that they do not have before taking the breathing test. You can do it for yourself to compare the signs of the table below. Note that you should have a glass of sugar juice next to you to drink when you have strange signs because it is the signs caused by hypoglycemia when you blow out:

- Blow out quickly, strongly and deeply by mouth

- Blow out slowly, gently and deeply by mouth

Table 5: Effect of different breathing on the blood pressure, glycemia and metabolism of the body.

Effect of different breathing on the blood pressure, glycemia, and metabolism of the body.
A. Quick, strong and deep breathing in respiration therapy
Experiments of quick, strong and deep breathing in respiration therapy
Group one: blow out quickly, strongly and deeply by mouth

for 5 minutes. This will burn out glucose quickly so that people started to yawn and the feeling of vertigo, dizziness, and the pain, stiffness, and numbness, in the face and the body's parts after five or ten minutes of practicing.

If they have back pain and neck pain before, their pain will become severer when taking deep and fast breathing in and out

Glucose in the blood reduce quickly. Systolic pressure reduced substantially and diastolic pressure reduced substantially.

Most of the irritating signs in the body were clear by a glass of sugar juice. If have any abnormal feelings, stop using the machine to check and drink sweet juice immediately. The more severe of the symptoms, the more sugar juice they need to take to clear it out.

A. Slow, gentle and deep breathing in respiration therapy.

Group two: blow out slowly, gently, and deeply by mouth for 10 minutes.

This will burn out glucose slowly so that after five or ten minutes, they do not have as many signs as group one.

These people only started to yawn and the feeling of vertigo, dizziness, and the pain, stiffness, and numbness, in the face and the body's parts after ten or twenty minutes of practicing. To stop these, we can do as slow as possible when breath out creating small voice like Oooo, or Uuuuuu; or practitioners can have a glass of sugar juice. To some extent, this deep breath is like smoking: breath in mouth deeply and slowly.

Glucose in the blood reduce slowly, and it was reduced substantially when participants start to have a strange feeling

Systolic pressure and diastolic pressure reduce slowly, and it was reduced substantially when participants start to have a strange feelings. Only some participants need to take sugar juice to clear out the strange signs.

By practicing and recording the signs, I see that blowing out will reduce the glycemia. If we blow out quickly and strongly, we will reduce the level of glucose in the bloodstream quickly and we will soon have the signs of hypoglycemia after 5 minutes of practicing. Our participants who had high blood pressure just blowing out strongly by mouth in five minutes had systolic pressure reduced 10 mmHg.

If we blow out slowly and deeply, we will not have signs of hypoglycemia after 5 minutes of practicing. This kind of breathing is similar to breathing in smoking. During smoking time: people start to breathe deeply and slowly by mouth. Breath The participants taking a breath by mouth slowly and deeply for 20 minutes can reduce both systolic pressure and diastolic pressure substantially, and their glycemia also reduced. Some participants had a feeling of reducing glucose level in the blood like yawning and the feeling of vertigo, dizziness, and the pain, stiffness, and numbness, in the face and body's parts. I confirm these feelings appeared caused by reducing glucose levels in the bloodstream because all of these feelings had been cleared out immediately just by taking a glass of sugar juice. These are the simple experiments that you can do by yourself. The deep breath of smoking may be the answer to why people who smoke tend to have

These kinds of breathing can be done by you and all other participants so that you can self prove the signs, symptoms, and applications? As a pharmacist and a trainer of respiration therapy in Qi Cong Y Dao Viet Nam, I see the immense application of the breathing in controlling glucose level and many metabolic diseases that we are facing.

Any higher amount or lower amount of ingredients than a balanced level will lead to metabolic disorders of the cells and dysfunctioning of the organs. Most of the techniques of Vietnamese Qi Gong is to aim at balancing the circulation system to the important organs and on the whole body. To have healthy circulation, therapists aim at the exercise that increases the mobility of the blood to the five important organs, nutrition, sugar intake, herbs, and the techniques removing the blocking points or trigger points. The poor circulation and the blocking points are the main cause of most symptoms like pain, numbness, irritation, stiffness. When the blocking points are near the blood circulation to the head, it can cause a lot of hypotension and hypoglycemia on the central nervous system. These points may around the neck, shoulder, and upper back. During the practicing, just within ten minutes, I could remove these trigger points and these central nervous systems disappeared immediately.

These are the exercise for Kungfu Master, who has a lot of experience in controlling the body, so if we want to follow this exercise, one crucial thing is that we have to drink sugar juice or eat sugar after five minutes of taking exercise or when we feel any abnormal senses during the exercise, these are the senses of hypoglycemia. To the people who have hypoglycemia or hypotension, they should drink sweet juice as soon as possible: sugar juice, coke, sweet juice.

Always place these juice nearby when start to take the exercise, and drink it immediately whenever you feel strange feelings: pain, numbness, tingling, vertigo, dizziness, short of breath, cold hand, cold sweating... it is the signs of hypoglycemia, all of these signs will be clear when you drink sugar juice. If these signs do not disappear after taking sweat juice, it means that the amount of juice is not enough.

To know more detail of the changes in the body, you should have the blood pressure machine and glucose blood machine to measure before, during, and after the exercise, especially whenever you have strange symptoms. Do not do this exercise when feeling hunger. Eat some things before taking exercise.

Chapter II: The relation between smoking, breathing, glycemia and the rate of the metabolism that reveals the effective way of controlling body weight and glycemia.

3. Body weight, smoking, feeling of hunger and glycemia

Try relaxed deep breathing for 10 minutes, then check the warmth of the hands and the glycemia, you will see impacts of breathing via the mouth deeply and slowly; which is quite similar the smoker inhale cigaretes. I have done this and let the practitioners to do it, the hands become warmer and the glycemia may rise a little. Mobilizing stored glucose into the blood stream make smokers do not feel hungry much, and do not gain weight while the people quit smoke gain weight and have more feeling of hungry.

A simple way to have relaxed deep breathing is:

1. Just try to breathe out via mouth or nose gently and slowly and as long as possible, when breathing out, pronounce small voice of OOOO or UUU or hahahahaha. By having this small sound, practitioners can have the breathing out longer 2-5 seconds than the breath without small sound. This can make the breath longer, deeper but the practitioners are not tired and do not have to try hard.

2. Do not try to breathe in, just breathe in normally. By practicing this, practitioners can have only 6 to 12 breaths in a minute.On average, people gain 5kg in the year after they stop smoking.

Weight gain is a common concern for people who are thinking about quitting smoking, even smoking consume more energy of the body, but the people who smoke do not have much feeling of hunger compared to when they quitting smoke. People quit smoking consume less energy but they have more feelings of hunger and start to gain weight even they are on the same diet. We do know that the feeling of hunger depends on the level of glucose in the bloodstream. When people have a high level of glucose in the body, they do not have the feeling of hungry or tired. But when they have a low level of glucose in the body, they start to feel hungry and tired. Before meals, if we let kids eat candy instead of vegetables, the kids will eat less because the feeling of hunger reduced.

People with diabetes will have a feeling of hunger, tired, or even cold sweating when it is late for the meal. This feeling is the feeling of hypoglycemia, it makes the feeling hunger and wants to eat food immediately. If the meals are not ready, they can eat some candy to reduce these feelings substantially. Cold sweating, trembling, tired, and feeling of hunger are the indicators that the level of glucose in the body reduced below the normal level.

In biochemistry, the main energy source of the body and cells is from carbohydrates. The body is a giant machine of countless metabolic reactions taken place all the time to create the energy for all activities of cells and organs. The main energy source for the brain is glucose. In a healthy body, most metabolic reactions to create needed energy for the function of body and cells are from metabolizing glucose, the other source is from metabolizing fatty acid. Many diabetic patients may feel dizziness, weakness, tremor, and cold sweating when they skip meals, most of these symptoms will diminish by eating some sweet candy or sweet juice. It is proof that the cells and organs of the body start to work poorly when the level of glucose in the bloodstream is below to the normal level.

Blood pressure, a vital sign that needs to observe in all inpatients, is the pressure of circulating blood on the walls of blood vessels. Most of this pressure is due to work is done by the heart by pumping blood through the circulatory system. Used without further specification, "blood pressure" usually refers to the pressure in large arteries of the systemic circulation. Blood pressure is usually expressed in terms of the systolic pressure (maximum during one heartbeat) over diastolic pressure (minimum in between two heartbeats) and is measured in millimeters of mercury (mmHg), above the surrounding atmospheric pressure.

During the time of practicing, reading the diastolic pressure can let the know the approximate level of glucose, triglycerides, and cholesterol in the body. When recording the blood pressure of the practitioners, most of the answer I got when seeing the number of diastolic pressure above 100mmHg, is that they have high lipidemia. Some recorded numbers that I found during practice is the table below that need scientists do some more researches:

Table 6: Variations of diastolic pressure during practice these techniques

Average blood pressure	Diastolic pressure when they are full	Diastolic pressure when they feel hungry or dizziness
120/70	80 mmHg	60 mmHg
130/90	100 mmHg	80 mmHg
These are the variations, temporary feeling that I recorded during practicing Vietnamese Qi Gong breathing.		

I found that to some extent, the changing of diastolic pressure of people vary around their average number. And the variation also has the relation to the changing of glucose in the body. During practice, when they felt tired or dizziness, I recorded the number of diastolic pressure below 10 mmHg compared to their average number. This finding can be easily tested for all readers with the kind of Qi Gong breathing, and need more attention from the scientists.

4. Effect of breathings on the glycemia in Khi Cong Y Dao Vietnam.

Respiration therapy in Khi Cong Y Dao Vietnam, an alternative form of health exercise founded by Master Do Duc Ngoc in 1980, Master Do is widely respected by many people for his expert knowledge of the ancient Eastern concept "Qi" or "Chi" energy. At its core, Khi Cong Y Dao Vietnam combines the idea of Chi energy with simple, specific physical exercises, which is able to stimulate the body to repair damage and regenerate itself.

Before the test, we check the blood pressure: systolic pressure/diastolic pressure. Then during the breathing, we check the blood pressure regularly, and when the participants said they have some strange feeling that they do not have before taking the breathing test. You can do it for yourself to compare the signs of the table below. Note that you should have a glass of sugar juice next to you to drink when you have strange signs because it is the signs caused by hypoglycemia when you blow out:

- Blow out quickly, strongly and deeply by mouth

- Blow out slowly, gently and deeply by mouth

By practicing and recording the signs, I found that blowing out will reduce glycemia. If we blow out quickly and strongly, we will reduce the level of glucose in the bloodstream quickly and we will soon have the signs of hypoglycemia after 5 minutes of practicing. Our participants who had high blood pressure just blowing out strongly by mouth in five minutes had systolic pressure reduced 10 mmHg.

If we blow out slowly and deeply, we will not have signs of hypoglycemia after 5 minutes of practicing. This kind of breathing is similar to breathing in smoking. During smoking time: people start to breathe deeply and slowly by mouth. During practicing Vietnamese Qi Gong breathing, The participants toke a breath by mouth slowly and deeply for 20 minutes can reduce both systolic pressure and diastolic pressure substantially, and their glycemia also reduced. Some participants had a feeling of reducing glucose level in the blood like yawning and the feeling of vertigo, dizziness, and the pain, stiffness, and numbness, in the face and body's parts. I confirmed these feelings appeared caused by reducing glucose levels in the bloodstream because all of these feelings had been cleared out immediately just by taking a glass of sugar juice. These kinds of breathing need much more research, it can reveal many effective therapies for many chronic diseases. These kinds of breathing are so simple that readers can do by themselves.

The differences in the experiment of breathing out slowly and breathing quickly makes me think that breathing slowly and deeply by mouth can help to mobilize the glycogen and lipids in the stomach and liver into the bloodstream so that the participants did not have the feeling of hunger did not reduce glucose in the blood and did not have to reduce blood pressure compared to the group taking breathing deeply and quickly. Smoking is also a proof for this kind of breath by mouth. Because smoking increases metabolism so that the smokers do not gain bodyweight, but the smokers do not have the feeling of hunger because each deep breathtaking in by mouth, help to mobilize the glycogen and lipids in the organs in the stomach and the liver into the bloodstream. The glucose mobilized by the deep breathing is more than the glucose consumed by nicotine in the cigarette so that they do not feel hunger. On the other hand, people who quit smoking will quit the habit of breathing deeply and slowly by mouth which makes them do not create chances to mobilize the glycogen and lipids in the organs in the stomach and the liver into the bloodstream so that the glucose in the bloodstream is low enough to create the feeling of hunger even they consume less energy than before. Just by taking a deep and slow breath by mouth several times a day can not only make the people who quit smoking do not have the feeling of hunger but also increase the metabolism of the body so that they do not gain weight after quit smoking.

These kinds of breathing can be done by you and all other participants so that you can self prove the signs, symptoms, and applications? As a pharmacist and a trainer of respiration therapy in Qi Cong Y Dao Viet Nam, I see the immense application of the breathing in controlling glucose level and many metabolic diseases that we are facing.

By joining hands together, we can connect modern medicine and traditional therapy, alternative therapy to help millions of people to have better health effectively, naturally, and cheaply. The indicators that can be tested by machines like blood pressure and glycemia are the firsts bridge to connect modern therapy and traditional therapy. Blood pressure and glucose in the blood are also the indicators that apply cheaply test whether or not any therapy using is suitable.

Chapter III. Self-removing the trigger points in the lungs to treat COVID-19, Corona, flu, flu A, cough, asthma, bronchitis, pneumonitis, and COPD

5. Practical view for self-finding and self-removing the trigger points in the lungs to treat COVID-19, Corona, flu, flu A, cough, asthma, bronchitis, pneumonitis, COPD, chest pain, coughing, difficulty breathing, tonsillitis, rhinitis.

Boost the lungs. to the illness caused by the virus, there is no medicine. But the health of the individuals makes a great difference. There is no medicine for these diseases. But right eating and exercise is the best advice for all. This is an exercise for lungs & removing trigger points.

Quickly and slightly punch on the back or on the chest under which there are the lungs, if there are places that the patients feel hurt, pain, breathlessness, causing the coughing or feel comfortable these are the trigger points that can make the lungs ill or pneumonitis. The trigger points I usually find are on the bottom of the lungs. We can remove these trigger points in the lungs by continuous punching on the lungs and the bottom of the lungs, which are the site of trigger points, for about 10 minutes each time. By asking the feeling of the patients and the sound during punching on the back we can know whether or not the trigger points have been removed?

You may feel like this is similar to postural drainage. No, this is better. The postural drainage technique makes patients feel lots of roughness on the back but does not make the lungs vibrate much. Punching on the back makes the whole lungs

26

vibrate, this will make patients breathe easier. Do this in the right degree can be seen as a massage for the lungs to boost the health of the lungs. To know how much the vibration of the vessels and cells in the lungs, just quickly punching on the table, and see the vibrations of dust and objects on the table. If we can punch with a quick rhythm, we can make the lungs vibrate most with the little effort. The more we do for patients, the better the patients feel.

Clapping removes trigger points in the lungs, removing the stiffness or rigidity of the vessels, cells in the lungs. Make blood circulate well in the lungs which helps the white blood cells to kill bacteria better. When the lungs are clear, it can take more oxygen and make people feel better, and stop the difficult breathings. The health of the lungs also impacts the health of the heart, intestine, liver, kidneys, blood vessels and the billion cells in the body, so removing the forgotten trigger points in the lungs we can make all the body in a good shape. Most people have chronic health problems also have problems in the lungs, just clapping on it, you can test the ideas. This can be applied and tested first for asthma, COPD, difficult breathing, and chronic coughing then using for Covid-19 patients

Cough is the body reflex when having some problems or stuck in the airway.

Cough is the body reflex when having some problems or stuck in the lungs, the body tries to throw it out by coughing. Punching on the back makes them have great relief. We may call stuck, dust, phlegms, constriction of vessels in the lungs as trigger points. If it is too much of trigger points in the lungs, patients will feel healthier in the chest, and difficult breathing. The cause of death by COVID -19 comes from difficult breathing, which reduces substantially oxygen saturation.

Epidemiology of COVID-19, the view that we may forget

- From the epidemiology of COVID-19, most fatal cases have many other chronic health problems like problems in cardiovascular. If they have cardio problems and vascular problems, I see the health of the heart has an impact on the health of the lungs. And the lungs also have lots of veins, tiny veins, which are the basic structure of the lungs - the proof is a kind of drug for high blood pressure treatment has impacts on veins have side effects is coughing. It means that the patients who have cardiovascular diseases also have lung problems. By clapping or punching, we can find it out.

- Do COVID-19, coronavirus, flu virus reveal that too many people have forgotten, untreated problems in systemic cardiovascular? Some of its drugs caused Coughing because the lungs contain lots of veins! Test by slightly punching/clapping on the back and the chest.

- From statistics, how can the young, the healthy men, and the females can self-prevent, self-heal flu caused by Coronavirus.

- Epidemiology of SARS may reveal that it is not the condition of the treatment but the health of the patients or the health of lungs, the systemic vessels decides the results of recovery or complication. Especially living in the polluted environment, people inhale a lot of contaminations that may deposit in the whole lungs and on the bottom of the lungs. By quick and slight punching on the back, we can make the whole lungs, bronchitis and blood vessels in the lungs vibrate with a rhythm.

- We do not have medicine for virus flu but we do know that by boosting the immune system, have good health can prevent and stop the flu. The complication of the 2019-nCov mainly on the lungs. Reading the epidemiology of the SARS, I sees that by making the lungs in good health, we can stop the epidemic of 2019-nCov.

- "Keto flu", the key for the flu, flu A, 2019 n-Cov, and the most chronic illnesses. Most of the symptoms of the Keto flu can eradicate by a glass of sugar or a bowl of soup. In other words, the cells and organs of people having a Keto diet or Low Carb diet are hungry, it makes the people on the diet have lots of flu-like symptoms. So remember to feed more the patients with nutritious food or sweet juice so that they can have warm hands, and the immune system can fight the virus, the immune system can repair the defects in the lungs and systemic vessels. Glucose is the basic energy for the whole body to have normal functions. Always bear in mind that keep level of glycemia at the level of 6.0 ml/dl when hungry.

- Preventing and treating Coronavirus, Covid-19 or Corona outbreaks lies in the finding and removing trigger points in the lungs and the whole body.

- From statistics, the same condition of treatment, how can the young, the healthy men, and the females can self-prevent, self-heal flu caused by Coronavirus. Not yet medicine cure viruses, asthma, COPD, Chronic bronchitis, difficult breathing, but the health of the patients makes a great difference. Most death cases had other diseases.

- The forgotten health problems: Covid-19 mortality rate, profoundly disturbing. It is not by the virus, but it may reveal the weakness of the modern medical system. It does not heal people, it just makes them feel temporary relief. It creates terms like chronic illness and asks them to take medication for blood pressure, glycemia, itchy, pain, irritation for years, decades, or lifetime. Many patients of chronic diseases have to take 4 - 5 pills for diabetes, cholesterol, hypertension, and impotent at the same time.

- They may wrong, they may create its own conflict, paradoxes in even one branch of medicine. Worst of all, they are come from the wrong belief on lifestyle, on the heath. When having problems with lipidemia, glycemia, blood pressure, nutrition in blood, they all taught to think of medication. Poor physical lifestyle caused a lot of health problems in developed countries, just google or Wikipedia. This is a fact.

- Many religious leaders infected and dying, even the high position in their religions, they even die when they are praying.

It makes me doubt God. Just a kind of belief and power of belief. If Darwin was right, then we have roots from animals, we do not need too much clean and isolating lifestyle. Look at the lives of 2300 years ago, 2000 years ago, 1400 years ago, 1000 years ago, 400 years ago, 100 years ago, if based on the modern standard of hygiene, the modern theory of diseases, theory in eating, drinking, all these people of these time should be dead because of a lot of diseases. So praying just have a little bit benefit.

- We may forget that the condition of living can have an impact on overall health and the immune system. I can only describe the paradoxes of living, paradoxes of David and Goliath, the advantages and disadvantages of having, pr of richness, of leisure/lazy lifestyle. Modern men may lazy caused they have too much and not think much of right giving, right taking. They may have a shallow view on physical and material life, tangible and intangible life, of giving or taking are the two faces of a coin/act/phenomenon.

6. Steps to help treat flu, flu A, COVID-19, cold, difficult breathing, coughing, asthma, bronchitis, COPD, pneumonitis, chest pain and flu complications.

These steps together can help to boost the lungs and other illnesses so that the respiratory diseases recovered faster and do not create any complications

A. Eat and drink first to warm up the body

The heat comes from metabolic reactions. To the weak, skinny, or chronically ill people, they need to take a lot of sugar juice to supply enough glucose for the cells. During practice, there are some learners who had chronic illnesses taken nearly 400 mg of sugar to have enough glucose for the cells. The glycemia should be maintained ranged from 6.0 mmol/l to 8 mmol/l.

B. Lie down and place an object on the lower abdomen, this will make the blood circulate well to the whole body

Lie down and place an object weigh about 1 kg to 2 kg on the lower abdomen. The object I usually uses was the bottle of water, a rock, a brick, or a handy bag. Place from 10 minutes to 30 minutes until they have warm hands and warm feet. During practice, I usually saw that the hand will warm first, then the stomach, and the foot.

1. If the hands and the foot warm, then do the third step

2. If the hands warm and the foot is not warm, these people can take more sugar juice then continue to lie down and put an object on the lower abdomen.

3. If the hands and the foot is not warm, even worse, the hand become colder and have cold sweating, stop immediately to start the first step to eat more and drink more sugar juice

There are a lot of soft tissues, soft organs and large vessels in the lower stomach so changing the vibration or movement of the lower stomach can make a great impact on blood circulation. This is the reason why deep breathing and abdominal breathing in yoga or qigong have many benefits on health.

C. Removing the trigger points in the lungs

We can use hands or rubber hammer to punch or clap on the back or on the chest. Cover the hand by gloves or cover the back by a towel to avoid redness on the back skins. Ask patients to sit up or lie down, then we clapping, or punching on the back and on the chest. Right punching/clapping makes patients feel better, calmer, and do not make them pain or the skin become red.

1.   Quickly and slightly punch on the back or on the chest under which there are the lungs, if there are places that the patients feel hurt, pain, breathlessness, trigger coughing or feel comfortable these are the trigger points that can make the lungs ill or pneumonitis. The trigger points I usually find are on the bottom of the lungs. We can remove these trigger points in the lungs by continuous punching on the lungs and the bottom of the lungs, which are the site of trigger points, for about 10 minutes each time. By asking the feeling of the patients and the sound during punching on the back we can know whether or not the trigger points have been removed?

2.   Continous doing these several days can remove all the forgotten trigger points in the lungs. After trigger points removed, clapping on the back just creates the normal feeling, no more the feeling hurt, pain, breathlessness or trigger coughing.

D. Clapping on trigger points on the whole body until having the sensation of roughness.

Clap on the muscle of the back, the shoulder, the neck, the nape, and the head.

When the practitioners have warm hand and/or foot, start to clap on the muscle on the back, the muscle on the lumber, the muscle on the neck, the muscle on the nape, and the muscle on the head; these are the areas that have many trigger points. Clapping on trigger points, people only feel numbness, continue clapping on it until people have the sensation of roughness or burning. The trigger points will be removed when people have the sensation of roughness or burning. Clap on those areas until all have a sensation of roughness.

Aims that therapies should aim

Always bear in mind that the exercises, right eating, drinking sugar juices and rhythmic pressing and suitable punching are to removing the trigger points and make the body in the good state which is shown in the hands and feet are warm.

1. The aim of self-healing is to have hand and feet warm and keep hands warm, soft, and a little moisture.

2. Keep glycemia at least 6.0 mmol/l when hungry.

Chapter IV. Keep the vessels at the optimum osmotic permeability

7. The vital role of circulation:

The blood is a red liquid, It consists of the plasma, the blood platelets, the red blood cells (the corpuscles), and the white blood cells (The corpuscles).

Heart, lungs, liver, intestine, stomach, lympho..., sexual organs, kidneys, hormones organs, brain, muscles, bones and all other organs in the body are interconnected by the blood circulation. All of the functions of these organs will be poorly when the blood circuation is poorly. Poor blood circulation may caused by blood clothings or trigger points in the muscles accumulates over time may make all the functions of these organs become weak, disorders and impaired.

In anatomy, the lungs, stomach, intestine, liver, kidneys, pancrea are structured by the tubes or tiny tubes which have structure are quite similar to the blood vessels. The fluidity of the fluid in these organs determine the blood circulation to the organs and the functions of the organs. To some extent, the blood circulation in the body and the functions of these organs are interdependent. These organs help to regulate the substances in the blood circulation.

A. The functions of the blood

The blood transfers the materials to all the body cells, where the red blood cells carry oxygen and carbon dioxide, and plasma transports the food, the vitamins, the salts, and the harmful wastes.

If the blood flow is a little poorly – or in hypotension state, it mean that the ceels will hunger for oxygens, excessive carbon dioxide and the many ceels in the body win hunger for food, vitamins and excessive harmful wastes

The blood protects the body, where the white blood cells attack the microbes that cause the diseases to the human, The blood platelets help in healing the wounds, and the blood keeps the temperature of the body constant.

If the blood flow is a little poorly – or in hypotension state, the white blood ceel cannot attack the microbes where the blood flow cannot reach well, so the microbes, impared cells, wasted and poisons cannot be remove by the immune system. The abnormal blood cloths prevent the white blood ceels and nutritions to reach to the cells and the harful wastes cannot be carried out.

The plasma is a yellow watery fluid in which all the blood components are suspended. It carries the needed food substances to the body cells, and it carries the harmful wastes that formed in the cells to get rid of them, The blood is a fluid due to the presence of the plasma which is a watery fluid.

Cells, tissues, and organs are interconnected by vessels and the tiny vessel which carries, systemic problems may appear if the vessel has the problems. Impaired vessels will make cells, organs connect together poorly. When the vessels are normal, interdependent organs: Heart, lungs, liver, intestine, stomach, lymph system, kidneys, hormones organs, brain, muscles, bones will be well cared for, fed and self recover.

The circulatory system, also called the cardiovascular system or the vascular system is an organ system that permits blood to circulate and transport nutrients (such as amino acids and electrolytes), oxygen, carbon dioxide, hormones, and blood cells to and from the cells in the body to provide nourishment and help in fighting diseases, stabilize temperature and pH, and maintain homeostasis.

The blood platelets

The blood platelets are the small cell fragments. It helps in the coagulation of the blood (the formation of the blood clot), So they help in healing the wounds. When the body is wounded and the blood exposed to the air, the platelets stick to prevent the bleeding and they heal the wounds. If the blood circulation to this cites poorly, the ability to heal the wounds will be poorly or impaired.

The red blood cells

The red blood cells are the red cells without the nuclei. They carry oxygen gas from the lungs to all the body cells, and they carry carbon dioxide gas from all the body cells to the lungs. Oxygen is the vital element of metabolic reaction in the cells which generates energy for all functions of the cells, if oxygens are poorly, the metabolic reactions may become disordered.

The white blood cells

The white blood cells are the white cells with the different forms of the nuclei, and they defend the body against the microbes by attacking them. These may be poorly if we have hypotension.

B. The quality of blood can be found in blood test, in simple, practitioners can see the quality of blood by checking glycemia and blood pressure

In practice, we should redefine the blood pressure, it is not the pressure of the flow in the vessels but it is the total pressure that we can feel on the surface of vessels which is the combination of the pressure of the flow in the vessel and the resistance of the systemic vessels. So the blood pressure not only represents the health of the heart but also represents the health of the systemic vessels and the thickness of the vessels.

Blood vessels cannot function properly when inhibited by vascular diseases. One of the most common diseases of the arteries is called atherosclerosis. In atherosclerosis, cholesterol and fatty deposits accumulate inside arterial walls leading to the formation of plaque. This inhibits blood flow to organs and tissues and can lead to further complications such as blood clots.

The elasticity of blood vessels enables them to circulate blood but a hardened plaque in arterial walls makes them too stiff to do this. Stiffened vessels may even rupture under pressure. Atherosclerosis can also cause the bulging of a weakened artery known as an aneurysm. Aneurysms create complications by pressing against organs and may rupture and cause internal bleeding if left untreated. Other vascular diseases include stroke, chronic venous insufficiency, and carotid artery disease.

Most venous problems are due to inflammation that results from an injury, blockage, defect, or infection—blood clots are commonly triggered by these. The formation of blood clots in superficial veins can cause superficial thrombophlebitis, which is characterized by clotted veins just beneath the surface of the skin. Blood clots in deep veins lead to a condition known as deep vein thrombosis. Varicose veins, which are enlarged veins that can lead to blood clots, may develop when damage to vein valves causes blood to accumulate.

These vessels are like interdependent vessels in the body. It means that if people have high blood pressure, a kind cardiovascular diseases, we know that the vascular appear in every organ, if we just only use cardiovascular medication to maintain blood pressure to the normal but not think of healing others organs, and the systemic vessels are disorders, over time, the disorders accumulated that we cannot heal. Or in other health conditions, the vascular problems may be more severe. In other words, we cannot cure high blood pressure if we do not think of the health of the Arteries, the Veins, the Capillaries, and the Sinusoids.

- Why do disordered blood pressure, diabetes, lipidemia always go together?
- Why do some skinny people also have diabetes?
- Why do some skinny people still have lipidemia?

The main reason that we may forget that blood pressure mainly represents the health of the vessels. In other words, it represents the thickness and resistance of the systemic vessels. The problems may be in the thickness of the vessels because it determines the endosmosis of the vessels. When the vessels are thicker than normal, it may keep acid amines, glucose, and lipid in the vessels. Keeping lipids too long and too much, we have high lipidemia. Keeping glucose too long, we have high Hba1c and diabetes. We may wrong advice all people with high glycemia eat less and intake less sugar. We may wrong advice all people with high lipidemia to eat less lipid. I also see some skinny people who have diabetes eat too little compared to the portions needed for survival. We are wrong that we do not check their body mass index (BMI). If they have low BMI, we should find a way to help them take more food rich in meat, carbohydrates, and lipid to increase weight, to make them healthier. If skinny people are weak, painful, and have chronic health problems, if they are skinner, they may never be cured!

The complication of a diabetic is that the glucose is kept in the vessels and can not reach the cells. Too much glucose in the blood vessels can change the PH acid of the blood. And too little of the glucose in the target cells may make the cells suffer acute hypoglycemia or chronic hypoglycemia. Target cells are cells in the brain, nerve, muscle, heart, lungs, kidneys, muscle, bones, and eyes.

All the vessels are the contained of cells also, high glycemia may make the vessels cells lack nutritions which create not only the vessels problems but also lots of systemic problems

Injecting insulin to reduce glycemia is mainly by mobilizing glucose from the vessels to the cells. If the nutritions are kept in the vessels too much and too long because of the poor endosmosis of the vessels, the organs will hungry, weak, irritation, painful, impaired, disordered, or if severer, organs failure. Complications of diabetes mellitus include problems that develop rapidly (acute) or over time (chronic) and may affect many organ systems. The complications of diabetes can dramatically impair quality of life and cause long-lasting disability. Injecting insulins help to reduce glucose in the bloodstreams. The glucose goes directly into the cells as an energy source. In the body all millions of cells in the organs die and born every day, the newborn cells will replace the old cells. If we do not feed them enough with the basic food, the number of dying cells may be more than the number of newborn cells, it means, over time, the body has degenerative organs. Many hungry organs may rupture and press on the nerve and bloodstream which will harm other organs. More severe, some organs may failure.

C. The complication of diabetes may be explained that the cells are hungry for so long.

> The complication of diabetes are hypertension, heart disease, eye disease, kidney disease (nephropathy), nerve damage affected patients report pain, tingling or buzzing sensations in their hands and/or feet (neuropathy), joint and foot problems, infections of the skin. diabetes can cause a number of skin conditions, including fungal (yeast) and bacterial infections, skin spotting (diabetic dermopathy), and a variety of spots, rashes, and bumpy or oddly textured skin patches, cognitive Issues. chronic uncontrolled diabetes appears to be associated with memory problems and dementia in the elderly and may increase the risk of Alzheimer's disease.

Complications of hypertension are clinical outcomes that result from persistent elevation of blood pressure. Hypertension is a risk factor for all clinical manifestations of atherosclerosis since it is a risk factor for atherosclerosis itself. It is an independent predisposing factor for heart failure, coronary artery disease, stroke, kidney disease, and peripheral arterial disease. It is the most important risk factor for cardiovascular morbidity and mortality, in industrialized countries

We should find a way to heal systemic tubes, we should not focus on short tubes that feed the heart. Because the health and quality of the vessels of a body are the same.

D. In a body, all in one, one in all.
If we forget, we may fail.

If we still see the organs in the body are separated organs, we can never heal the diseases. We just soothe the problems with expensive prices.

If we still see the diseases, in the body are the separated diseases, we can never heal it, and we can make it become chronic diseases.

If we see the symptoms are the separate symptoms, then use symptomatic medicine to help, we can never stop the reoccurrence of the symptoms.

We should see them in the big picture, they are interconnected and interdependent to find a way to heal all effectively.

If not, flu, cold, flu A, Covid-19, stress can harm severely lots of chronic people, weak people.

Poor blood circulation to the head can make cold forehead, insomnia, headache, dizziness, vertigo, sinusitis, rhinitis, seasonal allergy

E. The health of central nervous system

The problems of the central nervous system may be caused by the stiffness of the muscles in the neck, shoulder, and head, which will prevent the blood to bring glucose and oxygen to the head, brain, eyes, and ears. The functions of these organs may below average, impaired, or failure. The symptoms may appear much severer during stressful situations when the body and the brain consumes a lot of energy. Normally, the brain consumes 20% energy of the whole body, in a stressful situation, the brain may consume more than that but not only the trigger points prevent blood circulation but also in a stressful state, the body may have hypoglycemia and hypotension.

Furthermore, systemic problems of the kilometers of vessels in the body make the blood circulation of the whole body poorly, in all target cells there are lots of bio-detectors to send the information to the brain and autonomic nervous system to mobility the nutrition and the circulation of the whole body. The disordered of the blood vessels may make vasoconstriction and varicose veins irregularly. In the nose, there are a lot of tiny vessels to warm the air, if the air does not warm well, the cold air will irritate the throat, bronchus, and lungs.

When the brain and organs in the body experience stress, or in state of temporary localized ischemia, it can create systemic vasoconstriction that creates many symptoms like cold hands, cold feet, headache, cold forehead, stiff neck, vertigo, dizziness, hypoglycemia or hyperglycemia (caused by glucose stuck in the veins, it cannot go into the cells, organs), and hypotension, or hypertension. To some extent, these symptoms quite similar to the flu symptoms. All the vital functions of the cells and body need oxygen to metabolize the nutrients into energy in ATP or Kcal.

Poor blood circulation to the head can make a cold forehead, insomnia, headache, dizziness, vertigo, sinusitis, rhinitis, seasonal allergy, poor functions of the organs, or organs failure. The best cure is boosting the blood circulation for the nutrition to reach the organs and discard the wastes well.

Forget biology, forget biogenetics, forget biochemistry, forget the immune system, forget the metabolism when there are problems that reduce normal circulation: Glycemia and blood pressure.

What is oxygen in the blood circulation? When we talk about the vital role of oxygen, we forget that the vital role of oxygen is to interact with glucose in the cells catalyzed by many enzymes to generate energy. The main source to generate energy in cells is from glucose, enough glucose is as vital as enough oxygen.

The circulatory, or the vascular system, is an organ system that permits blood to circulate and transport nutrients (such as amino acids and electrolytes), oxygen, carbon dioxide, hormones, glucose and blood cells to and from the cells in the body to provide nourishment and help in fighting diseases, stabilize temperature and pH, and maintain homeostasis.

The movement of the muscles helps the vessels and the heart in circulating the blood. The facts are if we spleen the normal right arm for a month, we will have a weak right arm and a little atrophy on this arm. It is proved that the physical movements have great impacts on the blood circulation and the health of cells and organs.

F. The constriction of the muscle cells, the narrowed vessels

Cramp often occurs when the athletes on fear competitions, it is not caused by lacking calcium but by the localized hypoglycemia and hypotension in the organs. The more tired they are, the more cramp they have. The solution for the tired is taking rest or drinking sweat water. Most of the beverages for laboring workers contain sugars and other additives.

Most of these symptoms and the symptoms of fibromyalgia will be removed or reduced substantially by practicing these three steps. Furthermore, during practicing, I saw that increasing the heat of the body and removing the trigger point, we can deal with a lot of health symptoms and diseases.

The stiffness of the muscle on the shoulder

may press the vessels to the arms and hands, which causes the hands' pain, weakness, numbness, and tingling – most of the symptoms will be removed or reduced it is warmer by better blood circulation.

Poor blood circulation in the stomach makes cold stomach, cold gastric, rigid stomach's muscle, and poor mobility that makes the foods stay in the stomach too long that it can be spoilt that create odors and acid.

Most of these symptoms and the symptoms of fibromyalgia will be removed or reduced substantially by practicing these exercises. Furthermore, during practicing, I saw that increasing the heat of the body and removing the trigger point, we can deal with a lot of health symptoms and diseases.

Poor blood circulation in the stomach makes cold stomach, cold gastric, rigid stomach's muscle, liver, pancreas, urine, intestine, kidney, and poor mobility that makes the foods stay in the stomach too long that it can be spoilt that create odors and acid. This can make the functions, products of the liver, intestine become disorders which will make other relating organs have problems. Poor blood circulation to the soft tissues may make people feel pain or abnormal sensation.

The chronic poor blood circulation in the abdominal may create heart diseases, lung diseases, liver diseases, kidneys diseases, and organs failure. The kind of diseases and the severity of the diseases depends on the degree and the sites of poor blood circulation.

The cold and abnormal function of the muscle in the vessels, intestine muscle, stomach muscle will also prevent the blood circulation and substances exchanging between the heart, lungs, intestine, liver, kidneys, and soft tissues, which will make these organs function poorly. We do know that we will have heart ischemia when the blood to the heart is poorly. These trigger points in the muscles in the abdominal if not being removed will prevent blood circulation in the abdominal.

The itchy often have in the dry and cold skins, by strengthening the important organs and making warm skins, chronic itchy will disappear.

The movement of the muscles helps the vessels and the heart in circulating the blood. The facts are if we spleen the normal right arm for a month, we will have a weak right arm and a little atrophy on this arm. It is proved that the physical movements have great impacts on the blood circulation and the health of cells and organs.

The stiffness of the muscle in the lumbar may make the lumbar pain and prevent blood circulation to the foot which causes pain, irritation, tingling, and weakness in the legs, hips, knees, and feet.

The stiffness of the muscle on the neck and the nape will prevent the blood circulation to the neck, spine, and head, which cause degenerative spine, headache, dizziness, tingling, vertigo, Alzheimer's & neurodegenerative diseases and vestibular disorder.

All in one

One in all

The health of cardiovascular impact on other organs

And the health of cardiovascular may tell the heal of other organs.

The health of cardiovascular impact on other organs. And the health of cardiovascular may tell the heal of other organs.

So that one technique to help one organs may not help. The body is a giant eco-biochemical machines.

Softness and warmness is the signs of birth.

Stiffness and cold may be the signs of unhealthy.

Where the chemical reactions need balanced biostatistics to happen quickly and accurately under the internal environment of the body.

In anatomy, all of the organs in the body are constructed by vessels of different sizes and glucid, proteins, and lipids combined together.

And the organs are connected together by osmotic vessels.

Osmotic permeability of the vessels will have systemic impacts on the health of all organs in the body.

The indicators of the blood test will tell us the state of the body and the osmotic permeability of the organs.

8. Forget biology, forget the immune system when there are problems that reduce blood circulation.

What is oxygen in the blood circulation for? When we talk about the vital role of oxygen, we forget that the vital role of oxygen is to interact with glucose in the cells catalyzed by many enzymes to generate energy. The main source to generate energy in cells is from glucose, enough glucose is as vital as enough oxygen.

Forget biology, forget biogenetics, forget biochemistry, forget the immune system, forget the metabolism when there are problems that reduce normal circulation. Quality of blood circulation simply checked by glycemia and blood pressure.

The vascular system is an organ system that permits blood to circulate and transport nutrients (such as amino acids and electrolytes), oxygen, carbon dioxide, hormones, glucose and blood cells to and from the cells in the body to provide nourishment and help in fighting diseases, stabilize temperature and pH, and maintain homeostasis

> Globally, the average blood pressure, age-standardized, has remained about the same since 1975 to the present, at approx. 127/79 mmHg in men and 122/77 mmHg in women.

The blood pressure is influenced by cardiac output, total peripheral resistance, and arterial stiffness and varies depending on the situation, emotional state, activity, and relative health/disease states. In the short term, blood pressure is regulated by baroreceptors which act via the brain to influence the nervous and endocrine systems. The main purpose is to give the cells enough energy to function well which varies depending on the site, situation, emotional state, activity, and relative health/disease states

Blood pressure that is too low is called hypotension, and pressure that is consistently high is hypertension.

We do know that blood the pressure is the vital signs, but we are taught that hypotension is so dangerous that we forget the danger of lower blood pressure. So that most of the therapists only afraid of hypertension and skip the dangerous of hypotension. Blood pressure is the vital signs of a healthy body. Blood pressure tell us the state of the circulatory system, also called the cardiovascular system, an organ system that permits blood to circulate and transport nutrients (such as amino acids and electrolytes), oxygen, carbon dioxide, hormones, glucose and blood cells to and from the cells in the body to provide nourishment and help in fighting diseases, stabilize temperature and pH, and maintain homeostasis.

In practice, I recorded: healthy people only have the feeling of dizziness or vertigo when they have hypotension or hypoglycemia.

Interruptions of coronary circulation quickly cause heart attacks, in which the heart muscle is damaged by oxygen

46

starvation and glucose starvation. Such interruptions are usually caused by ischemic heart disease (coronary artery disease) and sometimes by embolism from other causes like obstruction in blood flow through vessels. Cardiologists are taught well about the vital role of blood circulation to the heart so they pay attention very closely to the healthy of the coronary arteries. Coronary artery disease causes the blood flow to the heart below the optimum level. but the facts are all the living cells of the body need an optimum level of the blood circulation. Many tissues and organs are not as important as the heart, so we do not see immediately the signs of localized ischemic of these tissues. Poor localized circulation will make the localized disordered metabolism which will lead to abnormal functions of the organs, and the cells may die quicker than normal, withdraw to an inactive state, or speed up the degeneration of the tissues. If too many tissues and organs have poor circulation for a long time, we may soon have systemic diseases or severe syndromes. This is why the hypotension should be paid more attention than normal. Any number of blood pressure below the normal number will cause the cells and organs to work below the normal level. I have seen many practitioners who said they feel more tired, dizziness, fatigue, or weakness since recent years, but when they went for a check-up, doctors could not find any diseases and problems. After checking their blood pressure, I usually got the number below the normal number, the systolic pressure may be around 110 mmHg or 100 mmHg. This made I think that, if these people have these low blood pressure for years or decades, they will get specific diseases. It is just the blood flow to all organs and tissues are below the optimum level.

Table 7: The signs and the effects of hypotension.

The signs and the effects of hypotension	The possible mechanism
· Lightheadedness or dizziness.	Not enough glucose and oxygen
· If the blood pressure is	Severe lacking glucose and

sufficiently low, fainting may occur.	oxygen
· Chest pain	Not enough glucose and oxygen make the heart and lung have to work more, this causes the pain
· Shortness of breath	The brain stimulate to take more breath to get oxygen
· Irregular heartbeat	Not enough glucose and oxygen
· Fever higher than 38.3 °C (101 °F)	Impaired thermoregulation
· Headache	Not enough glucose and oxygen
· Stiff neck	Not enough glucose and oxygen make the muscle cells become inactive. These are muscle we use most of the time.
· Severe upper back pain	Not enough glucose and oxygen make the muscle cells become inactive. These are muscle we use most of the time.
· Cough with sputum	
· Prolonged diarrhea or vo miting	Not enough glucose and oxygen make the muscle cells become inactive or semi-paralyzed mixed with overactive
· Dyspepsia (indigestion)	Not enough glucose and oxygen for the cells act well.
· Dysuria (painful	

urination)	
· Acute, life-threatening allergic reaction	The reduction of the immune system
· Seizures	Severe lacking glucose and oxygen make the brain cells overactive disharmony mixing with inactive.
· Loss of consciousness	Not enough glucose and oxygen
· Profound fatigue	Hypotension is the vital signs
· Temporary blurring or loss of vision	Not enough glucose and oxygen
· Black tarry stools	Not enough glucose and oxygen for the intestine cells.

Changing lifestyle, adequate diet is the advice for most diseases

We do know the vital role of exercise, but what mechanism we have not yet fully know, I just want to sum up some questions and facts of health relating to physical activity. Hope that the right answer will soon be found by the scientists.

Preventive therapies and alternative therapies are to aim to make the metabolic rate at the optimum level.

1) Why exercise?

2) Why a healthy diet, with good nutritions and fruits?

3) How does lifestyle help?

4) Why Do Women Live Longer Than Men?

It is maybe because of the combination:

- Women eat and drink less than men. Most pubs in Vietnam only have male guests.

- Women have less intense physical exercise than men, so it makes them have more rate of fibromyalgia.

- Women have more moderate laboring work then men, especially in developing countries, these laboring activities may help to increase the mobility of the blood circulation, reduce the free oxidants and make metabolic reactions more balanced than men have. This may be the reason why women do live longer than men. Especially in Eastern countries, where there is the domination of Confucianism, Men have more rights, more benefits, and more delicious food than women. And the women still have to do moderate laboring work than men like housework, kitchen work, taking care of children, taking care of grandchildren. Eating less and working more maybe the answer for why do women live longer than men.

These are the review that needs deeper researches, some of the techniques carried by I can be easily tested by the readers and researchers and we can gain the results immediately. Master Do Duc Ngoc is profound in teaching and combining these techniques to get the best results. This writing hope that scientists can do more research to find evidence and prooves to combine all advantages of modern medicine, traditional medicine, traditional techniques and alternative therapies to get effective treatments for all patients.

Chapter V. The vessels are the basic structures of the whole body.

9. There are four main types of blood vessels that each play their own role:

Table 8: There are four main types of blood vessels that each play their own role:

	Artery	Vein	Capillary	Sinusoids
Function	It carried oxygenated blood away from the heart, except for the pulmonary artery	It carries deoxygenated blood from the body part to the cells except the pulmonary vein	It takes care of the diffusions of gases and nutrients from blood to cells of the body	Deliver blood from larger arteries to veins. Permeable and leaky to allow for quick nutrient absorption
Lume	Small and marrow	Large	Very small	Very small
Wall	Thick	Thin	Very thin	Very thin
Other features	Presence of muscular walls Largest artery -	Presence of valve to avoid blackflow of blood	Smei permeable walls for the transportation of gases and nutrients	Located within the liver, spleen, and bone marrow

	aorta			

Structure of the blood vessels

The arteries and veins have three layers. The middle layer is thicker in the arteries than it is in the veins:

• **The inner layer**, tunica intima, is the thinnest layer. It is a single layer of flat cells (simple squamous epithelium) glued by a polysaccharide intercellular matrix, surrounded by a thin layer of subendothelial connective tissue interlaced with a number of circularly arranged elastic bands called the internal elastic lamina. A thin membrane of elastic fibers in the tunica intima run parallel to the vessel.

• **The middle layer tunica media** is the thickest layer in arteries. It consists of circularly arranged elastic fiber, connective tissue, polysaccharide substances, the second and third layer are separated by another thick elastic band called external elastic lamina. The tunica media may (especially in arteries) be rich in vascular smooth muscle, which controls the caliber of the vessel. Veins don't have the external elastic lamina, but only an internal one. The tunica media is thicker in the arteries rather than the veins.

• **The outer layer** is the tunica adventitia and the thickest layer in veins. It is entirely made of connective tissue. It also contains nerves that supply the vessel as well as nutrient capillaries (vasa vasorum) in the larger blood vessels.

Capillaries consist of a single layer of endothelial cells with a supporting subendothelium consisting of a basement membrane and connective tissue. When blood vessels connect to form a region of diffuse vascular supply it is called an anastomosis. Anastomoses provide critical alternative routes for blood to flow in case of blockages. Leg veins have valves which prevent backflow of the blood being pumped against gravity by the surrounding muscles.

10. Hormones and acts of medication on vessels

Most mordern medicines created by mimic the mechanism adrenalin and noradrenalin, the hormones of parasympathetic nervous system, have effects of vasoconstriction on the tubes of the body. The systemic effect of adrenalin are the proves that all organs and systems contructed by vessels and connect toghether by the vessels. In details, vessels are contructed by diff. The sympathetic nervous system is part of the autonomic nervous system, an extensive network of neurons that regulate the body's involuntary processes. Specifically, the sympathetic nervous system controls aspects of the body related to the flight-or-fight response, such as mobilizing fat reserves, increasing the heart rate, and releasing adrenaline. When the entire SNS is activated, there is a cascade of reactions from all the organ systems of the body, which prepare the individual to deal with an emergency. This includes an increase in heart rate, bronchial dilation, increase in cardiac output, and dilation of pupils. All of these reactions are directed towards heightened awareness and preparation to combat danger.

Blood circulation is preferentially targeted towards skeletal muscle, with a reduction in blood flow towards non-essential organs. Therefore, there is vasoconstriction in the gastrointestinal tract and skin, and compensatory piloerection to allow the body to remain warm. While it could be a short-lived physical danger that you have to either fight or escape from, the SNS could also be activated in response to long-term psychological or emotional stress.

Table 9: Side effects of three stress chemicals

Side effects of three chemicals creating stress			
Adrenalin	**Norepinephrine**	**Mild side effects Cortisol**	**Serious side effects cortisol**
Sweating	Pain, burning	Acne, dry skin, or thinning skin	Vision problems
Nausea and vomiting	Numbness, weakness, or cold	Bruising or discoloration of skin	Swelling
Pale skin	Slow or uneven heart rate	Insomnia	Rapid weight gain
Feeling short of breath	Trouble breathing	Mood changes	Shortness of breath
Dizziness	Vision, speech, or balance difficulties	Increased sweating	Severe depression or unusual thoughts or behaviors
Weakness or tremors	Blue lips or fingernails	Headache	Seizures
Headache	Spotted skin	Dizziness	Bloody or tarry stools
Feeling of nervousness or anxiousness		Nausea, stomach pain	Coughing up blood
High blood pressure symptoms: severe headache, blurred vision, buzzing in your ears, anxiety, confusion, chest pain, shortness of breath, uneven heartbeat, seizure			Symptoms of pancreatitis: pain in your upper stomach that spreads to your back; nausea and vomiting; or fast heart rate

| | | Low potassium |
| | | Dangerously high blood pressure |

Functions of blood, to have the normal funtions of the blood, remove all trigger points in the vessels. The trigger points maybe are the blood cloths, the atherosclerosis and the abnormal vassocontriction. To know whether or not there are trigger points in the vessels that connect the organs to other ograns, or in the organs, using suitalbe forces to see the feelings are normal or abnormal. Just quickly and slight clapping on the back, neck, legs, head and face, if there is feeling of roughness or normal, it mean there is no trigger points, if there are the feeling like pain, percing, numbness, irritation, hot, confortable, there may have lots of the trigger points. To the soft organs in the abdonimals or muscles, just or pressing on it by finger or thumb, if it is soft and normal, it means there is no trigger points, if it is hard, stiff, pain, percing, irritation, it means there are a lot of trigger points.

- Transportation : It transports the digested food substances , waste nitrogenous compounds , hormones and some enzymes (active or inactive) through the plasma , It transports O2 and CO2.
- Controlling : It controls the processes of metabolism , It keeps the body temperature at 37° C , It regulates the internal environment (homeostasis) such as osmotic potential , amount of water and pH in the tissues .
- Protection : It protects the body against the microbes and pathogenic organisms through the immunity involving the lymphatic system, It protects the blood itself against the bleeding by the formation of blood clot.

Stress and some asympathetic medication can have impacts on the vasocotriction of the vessels, which may create impacts on the functions of the vessels

Blood Pressure

The blood is a viscous liquid which circulates within the arteries and veins smoothly by the process of heartbeats , but to pass within the microscopic blood capillaries , it needs pressure. The maximum blood pressure is measured as the ventricles contract and the largest blood pressure is measured in the arteries nearer to the heart. The minimum blood pressure is measured as the ventricles relax and the blood pressure in the venules is very low (about 10 mm Hg) , This pressure is not sufficient to move the blood back to the heart , So , the returning of blood to the heart depends on :

The skeletal muscles near the veins : when these muscles contract , they put a pressure on the collapsible walls of veins and the blood contained in these vessels, so if the skeletal muscles too weak, it cannot help the blood circution. If the skeletons muscles are too stiff (in spasm) it may block blood circulation. So the health of the skeletal muscle and the trigger points in the muscles impact the localized blood circulation and systemic blood circulation. Valves of veins : that prevent the backward flow of blood. Valves of veins need enough food to function well. If the muscles are stiff, the valves may too stiff to control blood flow.

11. Forget medicines, forget modern techniques if cutting the energy source for the cells

What is oxygen in the blood circulation? When we talk about the vital role of oxygen, we forget that the vital role of oxygen is to interact with glucose in the cells catalyzed by many enzymes to generate energy. The main source to generate energy in cells is from glucose, enough glucose is as vital as enough oxygen.

A. Cells with metabolic reactions are the basic structure of all tissues and organs

Table 10: Catabolic reactions

Substrate + Oxy + Enzyme = Product + H_2O + Energy (ATP/heat) + Enzyme

These are the factors that I withdraw from inorganic reactions, organic reactions, and intercellular metabolic reactions catalyzed by enzymes.

Table 11: The factors that impact the catabolic reactions in the body

The factors that impact the catabolic reactions in the body: the cell, the reactions, the environment, and the whole body.
Factor 1: Concentration of Enzyme
Factor 2: Concentration of Substrate from digested foods
Factor 3: Concentration of Oxy
Factor 4: Concentration of products

Factor 5: Mobility of blood circulation or the mobility of fluid in the cells and around the tissues.
Factor 6: The state of the solution: homogeneous or inhomogeneous
Factor 7: Temperature: When two reactants are in the same fluid phase, their particles collide to have a reaction. If the reactants are uniformly dispersed in a single homogeneous, then the number of collisions per unit time depends on concentration and temperature.
Factor 8: PH of the environment.
Factor 9: Effect of Activators or cofactors. Some of the enzymes require certain inorganic metallic cations, like $Mg2+$, $Mn2+$, $Zn2+$, $Ca2+$, $Co2+$, $Cu2+$, $Na+$, $K+$, etc., for their optimum activity.
Factor 10: Some of the properties in this category are the state of matter, molecular size, bond type, and bond strength. - State of Matter - Bond Type - Bond Strength - Number of Bonds/Molecular Size

B. Hypoglycemia and hypothermia

Glycemia and temperature of specific tissues is crucial for the functions of the tissues, in practice, traditional therapist always feel the cold or low temperature in the pain legs, pain arm, or irritational stomach. It is the signs that abnormal areas temperature links to physical pain. If they check the blood glucose in the finger of the healthy hand and the finger of the tingling hand, they can see that there is a variation of these two numbers. These numbers are not the same even we do at the same time and to the same people. It is because of localized knots can prevent blood circulation.

When the body's ability to thermoregulate becomes hindered and is left untreated, organ failure is imminent. Blood flow will be reduced, leading to ischemia, and, ultimately, multiple organ failures.

Table 12: The signs and the effects of hypoglycemia

The signs and the effects of hypoglycemia		
Sympathetic nervous system	**Central nervous system**	
Produced by the counterregulatory hormones	Abnormal thinking, impaired judgment	Difficulty speaking, slurred speech
Shakiness, anxiety, nervousness	Nonspecific dysphoria, moodiness, depression, crying, exaggerated concerns	Ataxia, incoordination, sometimes mistaken for drunkenness
Palpitations, tachycardia	Feeling of numbness, pins and needles (paresthesia)	Focal or general motor deficit, paralysis, hemiparesis
Sweating	Negativism, irritability, belligerence, combativeness, rage	Headache
Pallor, coldness, clamminess	Personality change, emotional lability	Stupor, coma, abnormal breathing
Dilated pupils (mydriasis)	Fatigue, weakness, apathy, lethargy,	Generalized or focal seizures

	daydreaming, sleep	
Hunger, borborygmus	Confusion, memory loss, lightheadedness or dizziness, delirium	Abnormal thinking, impaired judgment
Nausea, vomiting, abdominal discomfort	Staring, glassy look, blurred vision, double vision	Nonspecific dysphoria, moodiness, depression, crying, exaggerated concerns
Headache	Flashes of light in the field of vision	Feeling of numbness, pins, and needles (paresthesia)
Shakiness, dysphoria. Significant hypoglycemia appears to increase the risk of cardiovascular disease	Automatic behavior, also known as automatism	Negativism, irritability, belligerence, combativeness, rage

Hypoglycemic symptoms can also occur when one is sleeping. Examples of symptoms during sleep can include damp bed sheets or clothes from perspiration. Having nightmares or the act of crying out can be a sign of hypoglycemia. Once the individual is awake they may feel tired, irritable, or confused and these may be signs of hypoglycemia as well. What if localized hypoglycemia, localized hypotension appears in the brain, and other tissues of the body for years or even the decades? I did record glycemia, temperature, and stiffness of the pain, numbness areas, the recorded results are much different from the normal areas of the same body. And when practitioners take sugar juice with suitable exercise, I did see when the localized glycemia, localized temperature back to normal, most of the pain and numbness disappeared.

Long-term effects of hypoglycemia may lead to permanent brain damage. The longterm effects of diabetes show the results that cells, organs, and tissues are under severe degeneration for years. It has been frequently found that those type 1 diabetics found "dead in bed" in the morning after suspected severe hypoglycemia had some underlying coronary pathology that led to an induced fatal heart attack.

C. Hypothermia

Hypoglycemia is also found in many people with hypothermia, as hypothermia, may be a result of hypoglycemia. The distribution of temperature in the body will lead us to know where the cells may suffer hypoglycemia and low temperature. The level of sugar in the blood is like the level of supplying energy for the billions of cells and organs function normally. Body temperature is also maintained by the function of the body cells. The whole body is a big biologic machine that all of the activities of the cells in the body are belong to the energy supplied by the reaction that control by enzymes and these enzymes are very sensitive to the changing of the temperature.

Table 13: The signs and the effects of hypothermia

The signs and the effects of hypothermia		
Mild	Moderate	Severe
With sympathetic nervous system	Mental status	Cold

excitation.	changes such as amnesia.	
Shivering	Confusion	No shivering
High blood pressure	Slurred speech	Hallucinations
Fast heart rate	Decreased reflexes	Inflamed skin
Fast respiratory rate	Loss of fine motor skills.	Pulmonary edema
Contraction of blood vessels	Mental status changes such as amnesia	Lack of reflexes
Increased urine production due to cold		Fixed dilated pupils
Mental confusion		Low blood pressure
Liver dysfunction may also be present		Physiological systems falter and heart rate, respiratory rate, and blood pressure all decrease.
		Pulse and respiration rates decrease
		Fast heart rates: ventricular tachycardia, atrial fibrillation

The circulatory or the vascular system is an organ system that permits blood to circulate and transport nutrients, oxygen, carbon dioxide, hormones, glucose and blood cells to and from the cells in the body to provide nourishment and help in fighting diseases, stabilize temperature and pH, and maintain homeostasis.

The blood pressure is influenced by cardiac output, total peripheral resistance, and arterial stiffness and varies depending on the situation, emotional state, activity, and relative health/disease states. In the short term, blood pressure is regulated by baroreceptors which act via the brain to influence the nervous and endocrine systems. The main purpose is to give the cells enough energy to function well which varies depending on the site, situation, emotional state, activity, and relative health/disease states

Blood pressure that is too low is called hypotension, and pressure that is consistently high is hypertension. In practice, I recorded: healthy people only have the feeling of dizziness or vertigo when they have hypotension or hypoglycemia.

12. Let the body to remove trigger point and balance metabolic reactions

Self-healing with right eating, right drinking sugar juice, and doing some of the exercises that can put the body in good state, the body can self-heal the defects and self-remove trigger points magically. To put the body in good state, we need to pay attention to the organs in the chest and abdomem which regulate most of ingredients in the blood stream.

The stomach, a place where digestion, absorption, and elimination has taken place, should be in a good state.

- In Vietnam, we are told to put a small blanket across the stomach of the kids during the sleep to make them sleep well and not ill.

- In traditional, when people have cold stomach pain, we are told to rub the topical hot medical ointments, drink sweet ginger juice, or massage the stomach.

- About laughing: why laughing has good effects on health? Happiness and moving all organs in the stomach. It is like to make all the organs in the stomach upsidedown. If we make the fake laugh, we do not get the result as the real laugh. If we just feel joy but not laughing, we do not get a good impact on health as a real laugh.

· These facts and the experience make I think of the vital role of blood circulation in health and chronic illness. Poor blood circulation may come from the blocking points in the vessels or from low blood pressure or low blood glucose. In the body, all the billions of cells of all body systems need the energy to have normal functions; which is mainly generated from metabolizing glucose. When the cells hunger for glucose, it can start to use structure stored glucose or stored lipids or polysaccharides or structure lipid or structure protein. To take stored glucose, the body needs good blood circulation and right body temperature. The people with chronic illness often have hormonal imbalanced – which need glucose as the main source of energy also, and poor blood circulation and disorder of thermoregulation. If we do not stop these disorders, these people may have metabolic disorders or metabolic diseases. The main energy source for the cells is from the catabolism of glucose. So any problem for glycemia and oxygen saturation will make the billions of cells of the body are out of balance.

A metabolic disorder can generate free oxygen and free radicals. On the other hand, the immune system is not in a good state because of the hunger for energy may fail in repairing the damage caused by metabolic disorders.

In traditional medicine, the pain mainly caused by trigger points, so all alternative therapies like acupressure, dry needle, massage aim to remove trigger points. In the metabolic view, I saw that the trigger points mainly in the muscle which presses the surrounding vessels of blood circulation. The signs of trigger point are pain, numbness, cold, or rigid. Poor blood circulation may make the target cells and target organs hunger for the glucose and poison by the metabolic wastes which are not carried out well by the poor blood circulation.

Glycemia, oxygen saturation, and blood pressure are mainly control by heart, vessels, liver, pancreatic, intestine, lungs, and kidneys. Any problems that happen to the heart, vessels, liver, pancreatic, intestine, lungs, or kidneys will make the whole body have the various problems described by syndromes or metabolic diseases. Only oxygen can not create energy, the body does not have stored oxygen we do need breath continuously. To have a good metabolism, the blood needs to supply glucose or substrates for the cells at the optimum levels. Supplying substrate for metabolic reactions depend on the blood circulation to carried stored glucose and stored lipid in the abdominal area.

The common advice for all people who have any diseases is the right laboring exercise like gym, exercise, yoga, qigong; and right diets.

65

Eating too much can make the body have too much stored-nutritions, this stored nutrition will create a lot of poisons for the body and have a burden for blood circulation and important organs. So the right advice to the people who have overweight is reducing eating and exercise more.

But the skinny and the weak people, the right advice for them are eating more and the right exercise. During practice, I saw that weak people have the cells are hunger and out of balanced; they all experience symptoms of weakness, dizziness, trouble in eating, trouble in sleeping, and trouble in studying.

The symptoms of the hungry cells are easily found in transient hypoglycemia in diabetic patients, when they late for meals or when they skip meals.

The most common cause of death in these extreme cases of starvation is myocardial infarction or organ failure. To healthy people, can easily feel hypoglycemia, hypotension, and the hungry cells of the body when they have hard labor work and skipping meals. The more they skip meals the more obvious they have the symptoms of hypoglycemia and hypotension.

If the chronic patients skipping meals too much, they may have cold sweating, cold hand, trembling, vertigo, headache, dizziness, or fainting which are described well in Vestibular disorder.

All of these symptoms can be easily eradicated by sweat juice, sweet candies, food or intravenous glucose transfusion.

During practice, I sees that with right eating or drinking sweet juice, and right exercise to increase blood circulation to all organs and cells in the body, and removing trigger points by clapping on it, most of the chronic symptoms disappear immediately in 10 minutes to 30 minutes of practicing.

Autoimmune diseases: what if we feed the organs poorly? The cells of the organs may die at the speed faster than the speed of creating new cells for the organs, we may have degenerative organs. The stressed and hungry immunes cells may see these degenerative organs and ill tissues as the pathogens. If we do not make the ill organs recover, we may have autoimmune diseases. These are the review and experiences that need deeper researches, some of the techniques carried by I can be easily tested by the readers and researchers and we can gain the results immediately. Master Do Duc Ngoc is profound in teaching and combining these techniques to get the best results. I hopes that scientists can do more research to find evidence and prooves to combine all advantages of modern medicine, traditional medicine, traditional techniques, and alternative therapies to get effective treatments for all patients.

2 simple Qigong excercises help self-healing

✓ Insomnia, headache, dizziness, vertigo, floating, Alzheimer's, chronic fatigue.

✓ Cold hand and feet, Raynaud, numbness and tingling in hands and feet, flatulent, dyspepsia indigestion.

✓ Diabetes, hypertension, hypotension, metabolic disorders, cardiovascular diseases, and varicose veins.

II. Placing object on the lower abominal

Before sleep, place rock or a bottle/tin of water weigh about 0.5kg on the lower abdomen for about 30 minutes, close the eyes, relaxed and watchthe moving of the object, you will easily sleep well. Having a glass of sugar juice or sweet juice if practitioner is skinny.

I. Relaxed deep breathing

Simple way to have relaxed deep breathing is:

1. Just try to breath out via mouth or nose gently and slowly and as long as possible, when breathing out, pronounce small voice of OOOO or UUU or hahahahaha. By having this small sound, practitioners can have the breathing out longer 2-5 seconds than the breath without small sound. This can make the breath longer, deeper but the practitioners are not tired and do not have to try hard.

2. Do not try to breathe in, just breathe in normally. By practicing this, practitioners can have only 6 to 12 breaths in a minute.

Always make the body have enough nutrition by eating and drinking to keep glycemia at least 6.0 mmol/l when hungry.

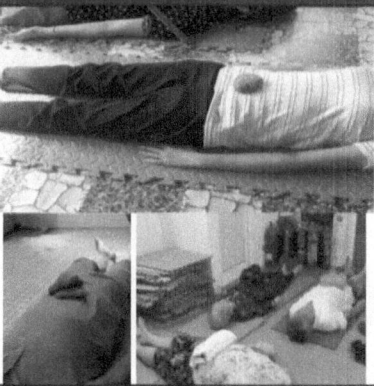

References:

1. Ebook"Awaken You Wonderful We" on Amazon
2. Review article: "The cause and possible cure for cancer and chronic diseases from applying Papaya leaf juice, baking soda, aspirin, sugar, temperature, Vietnamese Qi Gong breathing, exercise, metabolism, and traditional medicine."Van Duy Dao

These also good for:

• Asthma, Sinusitis, rhinitis, blocking nose, faceache seasonal allergy, chronic coughing,
• Pneumonia, tuberculosis, difficult breathing, COPD, chest pain, Shortness of breath, Cough with sputum and chronic respiratory problems.
• Cancer, Organs failure, irritation on the stomach, gastritic, and neurodegenerative Diseases, and Seizures.

2 simple Qigong excercises help self-healing

Daoduyvan.com   Awakenyouwonderfulwe.com

Picture 1: Applications of the healing

Chapter VI: Self-healing chronic diseases

13. Removing the trigger point and balancing metabolic reactions are the keys to fatigue, backache, headache, leg pain, neurodegenerative diseases, asthma, COPD, flu, fever, flu A, and COVID-19.

> Always bear in mind that the exercises, right eating, drinking sugar juices and rhythmic pressing and suitable punching are to removing the trigger points and make the body in the good state which is shown in the hands and feet are warm.
>
> During and after practice, to remain the results, always make the body have enough nutrition by eating and drinking and make the veins clear. To gain this state you can maintain these interdependent signs:
>
> 1. The aim of self-healing is to have hand and feet warm and keep hands warm, soft, and a little moisture.
>
> 2. Keep glycemia at least 6.0 mmol/l when hungry.

The techniques that help to treat insomnia, dizziness, hypotention, hypertension, nerve pain, chronic illness, eye diseases, vestibular disorder, diabetes, fibromyalgia, Alzheimer's diseases, flu, fatigue, backache, hemorrhoid, constipation, headache, leg pain, neurodegenerative diseases, asthma, COPD, flu, fever, flu A, and COVID-19.

> To the skinny people or the weak people, when feeling tired,
>
> - Stop
> - Then drink sweet water immediately.
> - If not have sugar, take rest till you feel better.

Just do from 5 to 10 minutes each excercise, when the hands still warm, you can do it longer. When feeling tired and having cold hands,

- Stop
- Then drink more sweet juice.
- If not have sugar, take rest till you feel better.

If the feeling of tired gone, it means the glycemia in the body is too low. You can have a glucose blood checker machine to know it.

Just choose the right exercises.

After several times of practicing, people with chronic illnesses can have diarrhea, nausea, or vomit, with the feelings of tiredness with hot and dry hands. It is the signs that the organs in the body in a better state push out all the harmful residues. Practitioners will be fine when all the residues are out.

Note that glycemia still reducing after 20 minutes when you stop taking the exercise because when you remove the knots, increase the circulation, the hungry, inactive cells start to act and take up much more glucose.

A. Eat and drink first

The heat comes from metabolic reactions. To remove the trigger points more heat the better. Just touching on the skins of the forehead, the back, the shoulder to feel whether or not the body has normal body temperature. To the weak, skinny, or chronically ill people, they need to take a lot of sugar juice to supply enough glucose for the cells. During practice, there are some learners who had chronic illnesses taken nearly 400 mg of sugar to have enough glucose for the cells. After two - hours practicing some qigong exercise, checking their glycemia, we got the number ranged from 6.0 mmol/l to 8 mmol/l. I was surprised that how the cells of their bodies were undergone.

70

To the people who have the right body weight or overweight and have a warm back and warm forehead may not need to drink sugar juice unless feel tired.

B. Lie down and place an object on the lower abdomen

Lie down and place an object weight about 1 kg to 2 kg on the lower abdomen. The object I usually uses was the bottle of water, a rock, a brick, or a handy bag. Place from 10 minutes to 30 minutes until they have warm hands and warm feet. During practice, I usually saw that the hand will warm first, then the stomach, and the foot.

- If the hands and the foot warm, then do the third step
- If the hands warm and the foot is not warm, these people can take more sugar juice then continue to lie down and put an object on the lower abdomen.
- If the hands and the feet are not warm, even worse, the hand become colder and have cold sweating, stop immediately to start the first step to eating more and drinking more sugar juice.

The warmth of the skin is from the heat of the metabolic reactions of the cells under the skin. When the cells under the skin hunger for glucose for the metabolic reactions, the skin is cold or dry.

During practice, I saw that there were some practitioners have the temperature in the hands increased just a little then it started to decreased immediately; this can explain that that glucose level in the blood starts to reduce substantially. I asked the practitioners to start to take more sugar juice if they want to continue.

All the physical exercises will increase the blood circulation to the muscle, organs, and cells in the whole body. The disadvantage of physical exercise make many people do not persist to follow because to gain good health from physical exercise, some people have to take hard physical exercise. There are a lot of soft tissues, soft organs, and large vessels in

71

the lower stomach so changing the vibration or movement of the lower stomach can make a great impact on blood circulation.

This is the reason why deep breathing and abdominal breathing in yoga or qigong have many benefits on health. After many times of practicing, I realized that by placing an object in the lower stomach, lying down and breathing normally, we put a rhythmic force directly on the blood circulation to boost the blood circulation. This exercise also helps people sleep easier and calm the stressed mind.

C. Relaxed deep breathing

The lungs take oxygen for the body, but the health of the lungs are interdependent to the health of other important organs and the whole body. Relaxed deep breathing makes the lungs healthier and equipped well oxygen for the whole body. Scientists and researchers do find out that the great benefit of deep breathing - a kind of exercise in Yoga, meditation, and Qigong.

During practice, when practitioners have relaxed, long deep breaths, they can have the hand warmer, feel much healthier, and soothes all the pain.

How can we know if someone has deep breathing? Just count that in one minute, how many breaths they take.

A simple way to have relaxed deep breathing is:

1. Just try to breathe out via mouth or nose gently and slowly and as long as possible, when breathing out, we can pronounce small voice of OOOO or UUU or hahahahaha. By having this small sound, practitioners can have the breathing out longer 2-5 seconds than the breath without small sound. This can make the breath longer, deeper but the practitioners are not tired and do not have to try hard.

2. Do not try to breathe in, just breathe in normally.

By practicing this, practitioners can have only 6 to 12

---

breaths in a minute. While the patients of asthma usually have 20 - 40 breaths per minute. The shorter the breath, the weaker they are. The shorter of the breath can make patients have more chest pain.

D. Clapping on the body to remove the trigger points until having the sensation of roughness.

- Clap on the muscle of the back, the shoulder, the neck, the nape, and the head
- Clap on the muscle around the temple bone, the nose, the eyebrows, the bones, quick and slightly clapping can make the born and mucus inside vibrate, open the contracted veins. You will feel well immediately when there is the feeling of roughness.

When the practitioners have warm hand and/or foot, start to clap on the muscle on the back, the muscle on the lumber, the muscle on the neck, the muscle on the nape and the muscle on the head; these are the areas have many trigger points. Clapping on trigger points, people only feel numbness, continue clapping on it until people have the sensation of roughness or burning. The trigger points will be removed when people have the sensation of roughness or burning. Clap on those areas until all have a sensation of roughness.

Self-checking before and after doing this by bending up and forth the neck, shoulder, heads, arm, the back and pressing around the eyebrows, noses.

E. Finding and removing trigger points in the lungs by comfortable clapping or punching.

We can use hands or rubber hammer to punch or clap on the back or on the chest. Cover the hand by gloves or cover the back by a towel to avoid redness on the back skins. Ask patients to sit up or lie down, then we clapping, or punching on the back and on the chest. Right punching/clapping makes patients feel better, calmer, and do not make them pain or the skin become red.

- Quickly and slightly punch on the back or on the chest under which there are the lungs, if there are places that the patients feel hurt, pain, breathlessness, trigger coughing or feel comfortable these are the trigger points that can make the lungs ill or pneumonitis. The trigger points I usually find are on the bottom of the lungs. We can remove these trigger points in the lungs by continuous punching on the lungs and the bottom of the lungs, which are the site of trigger points, for about 10 minutes each time. By asking the feeling of the patients and the sound during punching on the back we can know whether or not the trigger points have been removed?
- Continous doing these several days can remove all the forgotten trigger points in the lungs. After trigger points removed, clapping on the back just creates the normal feeling, no more the feeling hurt, pain, breathlessness or trigger coughing.

F. Removing trigger points in the stomach by pulling the knee to the chest and blow the air deeply and slowly

Lie on the floor, place the hand to pull the knee to the chest, during the pulling, blow out slowly and deeply when stopping the breath, loosen the hands for a while then move straight the foot to the floor, when moving the foot, just breath in quickly via the mouth, then repeat with another foot, do this for 5 to 10 minutes. If practitioners feeling tired too soon, try to pronounce small long Ooooo sound when blow out the air.

This exercise help to treat the problems of the organs in the abdominal. Self-checking before and after doing this by pressing the thumb on the stomach of people: right upper stomach (liver), left upper stomach (gastric), and middle-lower stomach (intestine, ovule or prostate), if it pain, there may be block for fluidity. This will reduce the trigger points in the stomach.

G. For varicose veins

Slightly tie the feet by rubber string or elastic crepe then walk on a single step or up the stair for 3 - 10 minutes each time.

Slightly rolls the elastic crepe around the calves, tighten a little more around gastrocnemius muscle because of this muscle have a lot of arteries: it will have a strong impact on the arteries and blood circulation when we walk the step. This help activate the blood circulation by making regular press on the veins in the legs while walking on the stair.

This also helps to make the blood pressure back to normal, reduce glycemia and boost blood circulation of the whole body.

H. For Insomnia

It is better to remove all trigger points, before sleep Place and object or a bottle/tin of water weight about 0.5kg on the lower abdomen from 10 minutes to 30 minutes, close the eyes, relaxed and watching the moving of the object, you will easily sleep well.

I. For eyes problems:

Self-checking before and after doing this by and pressing around the eyebrows to see whether or not there is percing or pain, if yes, there are the trigger points along the vessels that feed the eyes.

When the hands are warm, and all the trigger points on the head removed, just clapping all the eyebrows until you feel the sensation of roughness, your eyes will become brighter.

J. For hemorrhoid and constipation

Knit the anus 30 to 60 times a minute, do this for 10 minutes. This will make the anus' muscles and the veins in the anus become stronger which help heal hemorrhoid and constipation.

K. Loading energy, boosting blood circulation for five important organs.

Places 2 plates together on the floor. Stand with your feet slightly broader than shoulder-width, then twist the feet to make the toes move closer together, the toes make a V shape. Then bend the knees to make the 2 knees against each other, lower the body part, still keep the back upright, Stretch the arms in front keeping the fingers together then the palms up.

Stand like this for 5 to 10 minutes to make the body and the back warm or sweating. In twisting the feet, all muscles are much stretcher than not twisting the feet. This boost the blood circulation very well, stretching all the muscles very much so that the body will have sweating in just 5 or 10 minutes.

This exercise also used to test the health of the muscles of the legs, knees, and hips. If the blood circulation is not well, the practitioners may not stand in 2 minutes.

L. Boost the blood circulation and soften all muscles in hand, neck and shouder.

Losen all the muscle of the hands, flap or swing the hands and fast as possible, for 10 minutes. We can clap on the back of other people, or on the table, chair, in the air or on trees.

When loosening the muscle and flapping the hands, the blood will circulate well, the muscle will be softened, and well fed.

Do this can make the body warm and have sweating, it has a great impact on making ill people stop fever, reduce the pain and irritation. To the weak people who can not do the other exercise to warm up the body should do this exercise.

M. For nausea and vomitting

Try each or both of these exercise which can help soothe the irritation or force to vomit the residues in the stomach.

- Pulling the knee to the chest and blow the air deeply and slowly for 10 minutes.

- Clapping on the skin of the front neck until there is the feeling of roughness.

14. Self-healing chronic diseases.

A. Science of the Qi

Combining the factors that affect metabolism, the cause of most diseases and health problems with the Chinese traditional medicine, mechanism of alternative therapies, I assume that these are the factor to create balancing or the optimum of Qi.

Table 14: Balancing Qi

Balancing of the body can be measured by Qi. Balancing Qi may equal to all vital signs that are balanced. We can feel the Qi by the energy radiating from the cell, organs, and body by asking, seeing, examining, and touching. Balancing Qi means there is no localized abnormal signs and systemic abnormal signs.			
All these vital signs are interdependent with the changing of the intracellular and extracellular environments.			
Localized or systemic vital signs become imbalanced for a long time can lead to metabolic diseases.			
Blood pressure	Glycemia	Oxygen saturation	Body temperature
We usually use the general medical indicators to tell whether or not these vital signs are balanced. The measured indicators tell us about the whole body still in balancing			
For so long, we forget these vital signs of the specific areas, specific organs. Because of the vasodilation, contraction, blocking factors, the vital signs of the specific areas may be varied. Therapists of traditional medicine use all localized signs of the body, combine it to find the root of diseases.			
Localized hypertension	Localized hyperglycemia	Localized good oxygen	Localized hyperthermia

		saturation	
Localized hypotension	Localized hypoglycemia	Localized low oxygen saturation	Localized hypothermia

Then we will have the specific signs of lacking nutrition, lacking oxygens, lacking glucose, poor circulation. Just see the signs of hypotension, hypoglycemia, low oxygen saturation, hypothermia, hypertension, and hyperglycemia. The organs' functions may fluctuate with the fluctuation of these vital signs.

Result of right Qi or balancing of all vital signs: warm areas, the right temperature, the right skin color, healthy cells, and healthy organs, all function well.

The places that have abnormal metabolic can be seen as trigger points or knots. Trigger points, blood clots, or knots cause a lot of symptoms in the tissues and organs.

All these localized vital signs can go up and down according to the physical needs of the body and cells. Increasing and decreasing state alternatives replace each other.

If not balancing, we can have acute localized or systemic hypotension and localized or systemic hypotension. The imbalance makes the metabolism of the cells become disorder, this may make the process of degeneration or aging may become faster.

When traditional therapists touch the patients' shoulders. They feel bumps with the fingers that they call 'knots' or trigger points.

Fibromyalgia – a mild systemic disorder of metabolism that makes many muscles in the inactive state. Inactive muscle will make us feel pain, numbness, irritation. I remember the image of the cancerous cells light up when the mice were fed with baking soda by Dr. Dang Chi Van. I see that with a suitable impact, we can make these inactive cells will light up again, so the pain and irritation will diminish.

Myofascial trigger point: Activation of trigger points may be caused by a number of factors, including acute or chronic muscle overload, activation by other trigger points (key/satellite, primary/secondary), disease, psychological distress via the hormonal the system, homeostatic imbalances, direct trauma to the region, collision trauma such as a car crash which stresses many muscles and causes instant trigger points, infections. These are the factors that directly or indirectly impact on metabolism. The combination of some techniques in the next witing will show you how to remove the trigger points in just 10 minutes.

B. All of the steps in this chapter can use to help healing many chronic diseases.

- Warming the hand and feet and the whole body to reduce irritation, treat Raynaud, numbness and tingling in hands and feet, cold hands, feet, weakness and hands and legs

- Irritation bowel, irritation on the stomach, gastric, flatulent, dyspepsia indigestion, or pain in the liver, hepatitis, prolonged diarrhea, or vomiting.

- Insomnia, headache, dizziness, vertigo, floating, Alzheimer's, chronic fatigue and neurodegenerative Diseases, and Seizures

- Hepatitis, liver inflammation, pancreatitis, jaundice, chronic itching, eczema, constipation, and irritation bowel movement, chronic diarrheas, menstrual pain, Dysuria (painful urination), and cramp.

- Treating Sinusitis, rhinitis, blocking nose, faceache seasonal allergy, chronic coughing, pneumonia, poor sleeping, tuberculosis, and chronic respiratory problems

- Backache, neck pain, headache, shoulder pain, stiff neck, back pain, lumbar pain and nerve pain, numbness and tingling in hands and feet, cold hands, feet; the weakness.

Chapter VI: The cause and possible cure metabolic disorders and cancers.

15. The cause and possible cure metabolic disorders and cancers.

If the above practices, we should applying and do more researches to find the real cause and real cure for cancers and malignant diseases.

In practice, we do see some patients with maglignant cancers recovered from applying Papaya leaf juice, baking soda, aspirin, sugar, temperature, Vietnamese Qi Gong breathing, exercises, meditation, deep breathings, herbs, alternative healing, and traditional medicine.

In practice, I has seen many cases that have been successfully recovered from cancer by alternative therapies without using medicine. On the one hand, Some of them are recovered by Papaya leaf juice, some of them are by baking soda, some of them are by Qi Gong breathing or other therapies. On the other hand, the scientists also found that baking soda and raising body temperature also have a positive impact on cancer treatment so that physicians using baking soda and raising body temperature when applying chemotherapy for cancer. The question is how and why these cases are successful? The answer will give us an overall view of most diseases that we are dealing with. This is just part of my view and I have seen it had positive impacts on many cases. During studying the functions of the cells and organs, I thought: "All of these functions will poorly execute or do not happens at all if we give its poor fuels or cut important parts of the metabolic reactions. The cells and organs are in an ecosystem. All fuels or ingredients should at the precise biological amounts. Nothing more, nothing less. Too many sugars can be seen as too much fuel, it can destroy the body, most are described well with hyperglycemia, hypoglycemia, hypotension, and hypertension.

A. Possible results of metabolic disorders prove that metabolic disorders are the real cause.

These are the possible results of metabolic disorders that are proven by scientists. All of these problems do not have medicine but adequate diets and regular physical exercise, vitamins can help.

The metabolic disorder creates reactive factors like hydrogen peroxide (H_2O_2) hypochlorous acid (HClO), and free radicals such as the hydroxyl radical ($\cdot OH$) and the superoxide anion (O_2-). In traditional therapies, when to apply silver rings or silver spoons, we can see that the silver spoons have to change the color to darken. It is the result of reactions between silver and products of metabolic disorders. The facts are when the ill people usually have silver bracelet change the color into darker colors. These products of the metabolic disorder will damage to DNA can cause mutations and possibly cancer, if not reversed by DNA repair mechanisms, while damage to proteins causes enzyme inhibition, denaturation, and protein degradation.

B. Oxidative stress

Oxidative stress is thought to contribute to the development of a wide range of diseases including Alzheimer's disease, Parkinson's disease, the pathologies caused by diabetes, rheumatoid arthritis, and neurodegeneration in motor neuron diseases. Oxidative damage in DNA can cause cancer.

Radicals are only under controlled in a balanced state – Parkinson diseases

Radicals may also be involved in Parkinson's disease, senile and drug-induced deafness, schizophrenia, and Alzheimer's. The classic free-radical syndrome, the iron-storage disease hemochromatosis is typically associated with a constellation of free-radical-related symptoms including movement disorder, psychosis, skin pigmentary melanin abnormalities, deafness, arthritis, and diabetes mellitus

C. Neuritis is the general inflammation of the peripheral nervous system that may link to Parkinson's diseases, Leprosy, and diabetic complications.

Nerve injury is an injury to nervous tissue. Neurapraxia is a disorder of the peripheral nervous system in which there is a temporary loss of motor and sensory function due to blockage of nerve conduction, usually lasting an average of six to eight weeks before full recovery. Symptoms depend on the nerves involved but may include pain, paresthesia (pins-and-needles), paresis (weakness), hypoesthesia (numbness), anesthesia, paralysis, wasting, . and the disappearance of the reflexes.

D. Carcinogen

Carcinogen is any substance, radionuclide, or radiation that promotes carcinogenesis, the formation of cancer also may be the byproduct of metabolic disorder. When there is poor circulation, the repair for the DNA damage also reduced.

Is it genes or accumulation? We do see that genes are attacked by many factors and under continuous repairing. When the repairing is too weak, we may have damaged genes and a genetic disorder. Inside the cells, gene expression needs ATP and a series of anabolic reactions; these reactions also depend on the nature of substrates and nature of the environment, like PH, temperature, enzymes, and homeostasis. Carcinogen: this may be due to the ability to damage the genome or to the disruption of cellular metabolic processes.

After the carcinogen enters the body, the body makes an attempt to eliminate it through a process called biotransformation. The purpose of these reactions is to make the carcinogen more water-soluble so that it can be removed from the body, how can the body gain well this purpose when it is systemic or localized blood circulation.

84

E. Pain in many illnesses and in fibromyalgia

"Far away from the optimum level, all things may out of balanced."

Lacking nutrients, and oxygens: cells go into inactive state, cold or stiffness as the bacteria or the cancerous cells in the research of Dr. Dang Chi Van did to test the role of baking soda and cancerous cells. When in this state, the cell does not help the vessels in carrying blood, and it may press on the nearby vessels so that it reduces the supplying blood of the vessels to the target organs. On the other hand, these cells can press on the nerve tissue that causes pain or irritable sensations. The stiffness of the muscle cells in the back, neck, and lumbar may impact the neurons and vessels in the back. The compression makes the related cells, related vessels and related tissues function below the optimum level. In these areas, the rate of dying may exceed the rate of reproducing. This may be the reason why in many alternative therapies, we use heat to pain areas, or using back therapies on the back may help many painful conditions.

These disordered metabolic reactions create poisonous products, in traditional medicine, therapists called these organs to have negative Qi or negative energy. The oxidative stress, oxidative factors, and free radicals may change the color of the silver bracelet.

F. Other medical conditions that share similar symptoms as systemic metabolic disorders that need to have deeper research.

- AIDS: acquired immune deficiency syndrome may be a kind of degenerative immune system.

- Parkinson's disease may be view as degeneration of peripheral neurons and mild degeneration of central nervous neurons. Scientists found that Parkinson has a similarity to leprosy in genes. The reason maybe it has related to the degenerative of peripheral neuron cells.

- More research in ulcer prevention and treatment in leprosy is needed to better guide management of skin changes caused by leprosy-induced nerve damage. In many people who are exposed, the immune the system is able to eliminate the leprosy bacteria during the early infection stage before severe symptoms develop a genetic defect in cell-mediated immunity may cause a person to be susceptible to develop leprosy symptoms after exposure to the bacteria. The region of DNA responsible for this variability is also involved in Parkinson's disease, may be linked at the biochemical level.

- Alzheimer's may be viewed as the degeneration neurons in the brain. This is about Alzheimer's disease (AD), also referred to simply as Alzheimer's, is a chronic neurodegenerative disease that usually starts slowly and gradually worsens over time.

- May Alzheimer is the combination of severe brain nerve injury and mild peripheral nerve injury

- HIV makes immune injury? What is the role of nutrients and physical exercise to speed up the repairing of the injury?

- May the problems of diabetes: part of Parkinson's, part of leprosy, and part of Alzheimer's and all other degenerative of relating cells?

- Diabetic is a group of metabolic disorders characterized by high blood sugar levels over a prolonged period. Symptoms of high blood sugar include frequent urination, increased thirst, and increased hunger. If left untreated, diabetes can cause many complications. Acute complications can include diabetic ketoacidosis, hyperosmolar hyperglycemic state, or death. Serious long-term complications include cardiovascular disease, stroke, chronic kidney disease, foot ulcers, and damage to the eyes. Diabetic is simply seen as the high glucose in the blood and low glucose in all cells. When the problems are unsolved, the long-term complications are the results of severe degeneration of the cells and tissues because of the lacking glucose – an important material for metabolic reactions. Balanced diets and regular exercise play an

86

important role in preventing diabetic complications mainly because it increases the blood circulation which increases the chances for the cells to catch glucose.

PH acidity is also the by-product of disordered metabolism, PH acidity is not good for the cells and metabolic reactions, this is why baking soda may help many illnesses.

Chapter VII: The mind: stress and inner peace.

16. The brain with obsessed desires

The modified definition of stress: human beings have basic human needs described by Abraham Maslow. Anything threatens of satisfying these needs will lead to Fight and Flight responses. If people cannot change the situation, threaten, they will be the victims of STRESS AND STRESS HORMONES.

The limbic system controls the emotion, short-term memory, and autonomic nervous system. The cerebral cortex forms the function of the mind as an executive, cognitive, thinking with logic and imagination, control kinesthetic, hearing, and visualization. The cerebral cortex stores long-term memory and conscious behaviors. Human beings have a potential brain with unlimited power. The problem is why we get severely stressed and be the victims of chronic stress in spite of the fact that we are very smart and successful.

Human beings have been evolving a lot from our ancestors; we not only have the need for survival but also have many other needs; we not only obsessed with the need for survival but also we obsess with many other needs. Some groups of people have only basic needs; other groups of people have many needs. To some extent, the needs are expanding substantially in many groups of people with the advancement of living standards. The need to push and motivate people to work harder, longer, and more persistently. Owning for the needs, human beings have created many great advancements and developments for themselves and human kinds. On the one hand, people are the masters of the needs, they create many miracles with the noble deeds of noble need, the selfless needs. On the other hand, people may be the victims of vicious needs, selfish needs.

A. Human needs explaining by Abraham Maslow:

Abraham Maslow had taken researchers about human's needs and described the needs of human beings in "Maslow's hierarchy of needs":

The first needs are physiological needs, to do with the maintenance of the human body. If we are unwell, then little else matters until we recover.

The second needs are safety needs, about putting a roof over our heads and keeping us from harm.

The third needs are social belonging needs, about satisfying our tribal nature. If we are helpful and kind to others, they will want us as friends.

Fourth needs are esteem needs, for a higher position within a group. If people respect us, we have greater power.

Fifth needs are self-actualization needs, to 'become what we are capable of becoming', which would our greatest achievement.

B. Human needs explained by Tony Robbins

Recently, Tony Robbins has explained these needs of modern people in a much more understandable way. According to Tony Robbins, people have six basic needs:

The first needs are the needs of certainty - the need for safety, security, comfort, order, predictability, and control.

The Second needs are needs of uncertainty or excitement. We need variety, surprise, challenges, excitement, difference, adventure, and change. People hate boring things.

The third needs are the need for connection and love. As human beings, we all need to connect with others, and we all need love from others. The need come from communication, unified, approval, to feel connected with human beings, intimate and loved by members of the family and other human beings.

Fourth needs are needs of significance. Every people like to be significant. People need to have meaning, special, pride, needed, wanted, sense of importance, and worthy of love. They do all things to get and protect their significance. Most of the luxury products made to make people feel of significance.

Fifth needs are the needs of development. People need constant emotional, intellectual, and spiritual development. This need drives us to study more and do harder to make us develop.

Sixth needs are needs of contribution, the need to give beyond ourselves, give, care, protect, and serve others, to leave a legacy.

What do the human needs mean?

Most people have their own set of needs. With specific individuals, receiving rewards means that they receive tangible and intangible things that satisfy their needs. Receiving rewards will make people feel safe, happy, joyful, inspired, and motivated; receiving rewards make people filled with happy chemicals.

On the other hand, with some individuals, punishing these individuals means they will suffer the losses of tangible things or intangible things, which are the things they need to satisfy their needs. Being Punishment means bearing the losses. People perceive the actions of other people as punishments if the actions make them have the feeling of losses and the feelings of reducing their need satisfaction. Punishing make people have the feeling of reducing their certainty, their excitement, their connection and love, their significance, their development, and their contribution. These actions of punishment will make people feel unsafe, disappointed, annoyed, angry, sad, and extremely stressful.

At some stage of life, they have one or some needs stronger than other needs. With some groups of people, these needs are increasing. They need more and more. To satisfy these expanding needs they have to accumulate and possess

90

thousand precious things. If outside conditions meet our needs, it means these needs are satisfied, the happy system activated, chemicals of happiness appear in brain and body make us have good feelings. As human creatures, we want to have more happy feelings. The actions of animals are to satisfy the need for survival; on the other hand, human beings act to make them have a feeling of happiness. The drive of thoughts, behaviors of human beings is feelings - happy feelings. Collecting, accumulating, achieving, receiving, wearing only make people feel happy; they are happy when these things are satisfied with individuals' needs. All actions are to find joy from hunting, training, studying, kickboxing, playing, beating, killing, breaking, or suicide. People have a sophisticated brain than people can imagine, with memory, intelligence, and imagination, people do not find joy directly from the actions. They find joy in every action based on their perception of the actions. Memory and imagination make their perceptions have private meaning. These are two kinds of joy: short-term joy and long-term joy, or short-term gain and long-term gain. All animals' behavior is to have immediate satisfaction; they do not have the ability to think in the long term. All worthwhile achievements in the world are the result of long-term gain, the mind of human beings makes them direct the action to the long-term gain. The potential of the brain helps them accept short-term pain gracefully and joyfully on the way to accomplish worthwhile results.

17. STRESS MEANS PROBLEMS ARE BIGGER
THAN ABILITIES

What chemicals circulate in our bodies when we stressed? Many studies have shown that there is three main chemicals cause stress. These are adrenaline, cortisone, and norepinephrine. The three major stress hormones explained the "fight or flight" system that takes over us when we in a dangerous situation or when we are stressed. This was the survival system for our ancestors to survive well in a dangerous environment. This survival system does not help us much in a safe, constant changing of our modern society. Sometimes the constant trigger of this system can cause us a lot of problems. In our daily life, sometimes the small change in life makes a stranger, unexpected but safe thing happen to us but our survival system triggered. This makes us annoyed a lot. Constant of this activating can cause us fatigued, tiredness, and stress a lot. For example, when you received a friend's call from the office's number late at night, your body reacts so much stressful as if there would be an attack from a tiger behind.

According to Sarah Klein (2013) from Huffingtonpost.com with the article: "Adrenaline, Cortisol, Norepinephrine: The Three Major Stress Hormones, Explained", three major stress chemicals are adrenalin, cortisol, and norepinephrine [31]. Cortisol, adrenalin, along with nor-epinephrine is largely responsible for the vigorous and immediate reactions when being stressed. Cortisol is a stress hormone. In survival mode, the optimal amount of cortisol can save a life. Cortisol helps maintain fluid balance, increase glucose in the blood, and maintain fluid balance. On the other hand, cortisol reduces some body functions that are not crucial in stressful conditions, like reproductive drive, immunity, digestion, growth, and many more functions that are no need for the survival situation. A temporary increase in cortisol is very helpful for a critical situation. People will get many serious problems when

92

the body continuously releases cortisol. Too much cortisol can reduce substantially some body functions; which are the immune system, reduce memory ability, reduce mental capacity, increase stomach problems, increase blood pressure, increase blood sugar, decrease libido, produce acne, and lead to obesity and many more problems I will describe later.

In critical condition, especially the anaphylactic shock, physicians use a large amount of adrenaline, norepinephrine, and corticosteroid to save the life of the patients. Reading the mechanism of these chemicals will help readers understand why stressed people have signs and symptoms. Chronic stress leads to chronically elevated levels of adrenaline, norepinephrine, and cortisol, which are the causes of many illnesses and problems in children and adults like stomach problems, intestine problems, poor memory ability, poor mental capacity, and diabetes. We can know by seeing the increasing heartbeats, sweating, pale skin, gray skin, and the tension of muscle in actions, which has its own motive: vigorousness, suddenness, making noise, short and quick breath, non-smoothly action, and the stiff handshake. If you pay attention closely, we can sense or see these signals from stressed people. When people are angry or stressed, they will have the signals of stress are so obvious that most of their relatives can realize. In the stressed state, you will feel a surge of energy, which you might need to run away from a dangerous situation or fight against simulations. Stressed people tend to over-react with even mild stimulations from the environment. When people are stressed or peaceful, they can radiate the pattern of stressed energy or peaceful energy to other people around them. Dogs can sense the energy of opposite individuals in a blink. If you are under stress, your dog may stay away from you, lying quietly. Otherwise, when you are in happiness, your dog will go around you; a dog will play and make fun of you ceaselessly. Children can sense the energy from parents and adults more accurately than adults can. So that people can feel peaceful with a nice, calm stranger; otherwise, children will have the feel of stress with sad, negative people. After staying with stress, negative people, children may have some abnormal behaviors of stress. The mind of children - fragile creatures - can catch better and retain longer the visible and invisible stress signals than adults do.

Table 12: Effects of three stress chemicals

Side effects of three chemicals creating stress			
Adrenalin	**Norepineprhine**	**Less serious side effects Cortisol**	**Serious side effects cortisol**
Sweating	Pain, burning	Acne, dry skin, or thinning skin	Vision problems
Nausea and vomiting	Numbness, weakness, or cold	Bruising or discoloration of skin	Swelling
Pale skin	Slow or uneven heart rate	Insomnia	Rapid weight gain
Feeling short of breath	Trouble breathing	Mood changes	Shortness of breath
Dizziness	Vision, speech, or balance difficulties	Increased sweating	Severe depression or unusual thoughts or behaviors

Weakness or tremors	Blue lips or fingernails	Headache	Seizures
Headache	Spotted skin	Dizziness	Bloody or tarry stools
Feeling of nervousness or anxiousness		Nausea, stomach pain	Coughing up blood
High blood pressure symptoms: severe headache, blurred vision, buzzing in your ears, anxiety, confusion, chest pain, shortness of breath, uneven heartbeat, seizure			Symptoms of pancreatitis: pain in your upper stomach that spreads to your back; nausea and vomiting; or fast heart rate
			Low potassium
			Dangerously high blood pressure

READ FIGHT, FLIGHT or INDIFFERENCE SIGNALS

Hunger for human needs.

In their behaviors: if yes, they are stress. You only have these kinds of behaviors when you in stress. As you see, they lack social skills, they cannot talk: language is the product of living environment - as your native language and my native language; we speak it naturally without thinking at all. We are not born with our native language, so I doubt their connection with their living environment and/or the state of mind that they cannot or do not want to learn. You can test them with Aesop fables which they do not understand much, pretending game - they do not understand, interacting, communicating, or persuading. They are at the low level of this. For the official test: you can test them with EQ test, and Aesop stories, metaphors. All these low-level vital skills make them never feel safe, connection to the environment: it makes them stress. Over time, it makes the downward spirals that make them more and more lack of social skills and suffer more stress. Autism, Dyslexia: is the product of the environment, they are not born with its. When you know they are suffering from STRESS. You will see and understand the mechanism of meditation, NLP, hypnotism, Love, Caring, Touch, kissing, communicating for understanding.

18. The role of meditation to have a healthy, happy life

Practicing meditation regularly, people will have less emotional behaviors; they will reduce most of their greed and anger. Practicing meditation helps people gain the correct understanding of their body, feelings, perceptions, mental formations, and consciousness. Living with awareness, they have deep look at everything; they gain understanding. Understanding creates compassion and love. They can control emotion easily. Owning for practicing meditation, they can reach to state: the stillness of mind in the midst of changing world.

To practice meditation find a quiet place, sit on a chair with comfortable position, feet put straight on the ground; or we can sit on the floor, straight back, with our head, neck, and back aligned vertically. This allows the breath to flow most easily. Close the eyes slightly. For those who have dizziness hard to close their eyes can open their eyes and look down. We usually practice the sitting meditation either on a chair or on the floor. If choosing a chair, use one that has a straight back and that allows our feet to be flat on the floor. We sit away from the back of the chair so that your spine is self-supporting. If choosing to sit on the floor, sit on a firm, thick cushion to raise our buttocks off the floor four inches; thick cushion help us not falling backward; it can be a pillow folded over once or twice does nicely, or a meditation cushion. There are a number of cross-legged sitting postures and kneeling postures that some people use when they sit on the floor, choose the position that most comfortable for you. The main points to keep in mind your posture are to try to keep the back, neck, and head aligned in the vertical, to relax the shoulders in the picture.

Picture 2: sitting postures of meditation

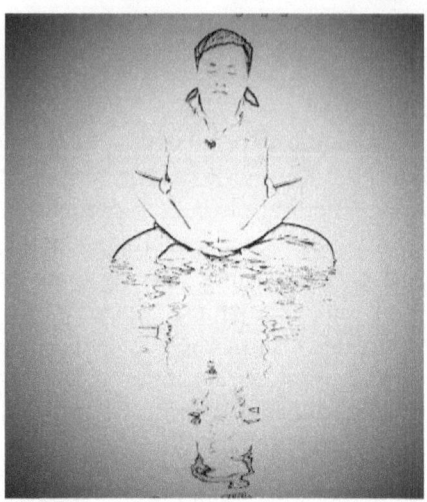

Before practicing meditation, people never thought about what was going on inside the body and mind. They rarely pay attention to the body, feeling, perception, mental formations, and consciousness, which appear and grow enough to make people follow their commands. With the habit of meditation, they realize all of these things still happen inside the mind are constantly changing things, they are aware of things going on and off; they get the better understanding so that they can know the time to stop, time to act and time to attach or detach. People can make a good decision whether or not to follow the commands, the conclusions, sensations, and feelings in the mind. They understand themselves better, and the understanding has given them more flexibility, freedom and peaceful mind.

Quality of life belong to the quality of the connection between beings, so do the connections of the neuron cells determine the power of the brain. All brain's parts active and work harmoniously during meditation. Mindfulness in meditation help the neo-cortex understands and establishes the connection to the limbic systems and other parts of the brain. Observing mind, body, breath, sensual signals and thinking but not chasing to the thoughts and feelings help us understand the mind, body, and life. During meditation, the cognitive mind start to observe the autonomic mind, the observation helps to create more bonds inside the brain. Owing to better quality and quantity of connection inside the brain, so that parts of the brain for the different function and billions of neurons become the identical brain. Good connections make the cognitive mind and autonomic mind work harmoniously. The more of practicing meditation, the more powerful the mind is. For any function of mind, all parts of the brain and neuron cells are synergic to fulfill the task. Scientists have measured that the brainwave of Tibetan meditation practitioners thinking of kindness is the highest human brain wave ever recorded; this brainwave is as high as the brain wave during seizure attack.

Meditation helps people live more mindfully, live close to the present, understand how mysterious life is so that they can sense the happy feelings. Meditation connects all the cognitive mind, intuitive mind, body, and environment together. Buddha connected to all other beings loved all other beings, and he contemplated to gain the highest understanding. Then all his life was to love, help, connect, give and teach needed people. His time may be the ignorant time of human beings but he had gained peace and stillness of his mind; he was the most content man ever. So that it is true to say Buddha is the happiest man ever.

A. Buddhism meditation

Thich Nhat Hanh told Buddha taught understanding gives rise to compassion and love, which in turn give rise to correct action. In order to love, it is first necessary to understand, so understanding is the key to liberation. In order to attain a clear understanding, it is necessary to live mindfully, making direct contact with life in the present moment, truly seeing what is taking place within and outside of oneself. "A person is a person who dwells in mindfulness. Life can only take place in the present moment. If we lose the present moment, we lose the life. He is aware of what is going on in the present moment, what is going on in his body, feelings, mind, and objects of mind. He knows how to look deeply at things in the present moment." Thich Nhat Hanh continued to recite the teachings of Buddha. If one makes good at present he need not care or looking for the future. Future is formed by the quality of present actions. So stop to pursuit the past, stop chasing to the future. Live closely and mindfully at present. Reading to this line, all you read one second before, one minute before and one hour before called the past. Do the moments perish? No, they all invisible embed in all parts, all cells of you. So if you live mindfully in present, you will gain the understanding to take advantage of the past and the future will take care of itself.

What is meant by "pursuing the past" and "losing yourself in the future"? To pursue the past means to lose yourself in thoughts about what you looked like in the past, what your feelings were then, what rank and position you held, what happiness or suffering you experienced then. Giving rise to such thoughts entangles you in the past. You may relieve the pain of the past, or regret the past that you forget that you are standing in the mysterious land. Losing yourself in the future means lose thoughts about the future, expectation and forget present. You imagine, hope, fear, or worry about the future, wondering what you will look like, what your feelings will be, whether you will have happiness or suffering. You may create some expectation in the future; you may be hurt or stressed of your expectation are not satisfied. Past and future only should use for your contemplation, for solitude but not for present living. Pursuing the past or losing in the future will distort your thinking, you may think you know everything or you only pick up the clues to prove your subjective judgments, assumptions or expectations. Your work, words, thinking will full of past and future events. At home, you will think at work, at work you will think and prepare for home or holiday. Staying with your children you may still relive the anger of the work, then, at work, you have to use the joy of playing with your children to bear the hardships of the work. Working like this you will never sense the joy of working, the invaluable of working. What a tragedy for the world when millions of people do not have a job, their desires may be having a job to feed the families, they may admire the neighbor workers. But they do not know that the workers and officers next door are tired and stressed because of the thinking have to work. Living with the success of the past or the victory of the future you will never see the mysterious around you at present. You will be slaved by desires and anxieties and lose the precious present. You will be exhausted from pursuing the past and future and losing of desires and anxieties because of the unwanted events in the past and future. Unfortunately, you may stressful and you will never really live. Mindfulness enables you to return to the present moment. You will lose your mindfulness and you will not be truly present for life.

> "Past and future only should use for your contemplation, for solitude but not for present living"

Mindfulness living makes you sense the joy, the wonder of living. Mindfulness living makes you understand life is so simple and life is full of paradoxes with intelligent people. When you live mindfully, you will remove all your assumptions and be open to new things. Mindfulness helps people know to detach with things, events, and phenomena. Art of selling has focused the mind of customers to live with the joy of the possessing in the future; the pain of not possessing; and the countless stories about what the product will make them feel. Customers will forget or do not pay much attention to the facts that they are trading in the present.

Mindful eating will make you sense the mystery of the foods, the delicious of the foods. Monks eat in mindfulness with simple foods. But un-mindful meal means when you eat you only focus on the unwanted things, unsatisfied desires, or any unwanted dishes on the table of delicious full dishes.

Never angry, sad or greedy people satisfied with the food on their dishes. Eating and all other activities of human beings depend mostly on the state of mind. Greedy people will never satisfy with whatever food, whatever home, whatever living, whatever jobs; and their powerful brain will taking the order of anger mind to make them feel right. It is so funny that they do not understand the mind, they tend to things that it is the law of attraction, and they are the centers of attraction.

Does mindfulness help people from suffering the tragedy of living? Be aware in order to see both the suffering and the wonders of life. Thich Nhat Hanh said "Buddha teach being in touch with suffering does not mean to become lost in it. Being in touch with the wonders of life does not mean to lose ourselves in them either. Being in touch is to truly encounter life, to see it deeply. If we directly encounter life, we will understand its interdependent and impermanent nature. Thanks to that, we will no longer lose ourselves in desire, anger, and craving. We will dwell in freedom and liberation." To dwell in mindfulness means the practitioner remains aware of everything taking place in his body, feelings, mind, and objects of mind; these are the four establishments of mindfulness or awareness. The mysterious of meditation that rarely people know, sitting in meditation simply just need you aware of body, feelings, mind, and objects of mind. Aware then detach to see its changing. Meditation practitioners will understand the hidden philosophy in nature and all phenomena, the philosophy of kindness, unconditional love, and compassionate heart.

Practicing mindfulness strengthens the ability to look deeply into the heart of anything. When we look deeply into the heart of anything, it will reveal itself. This is the secret treasure of mindfulness. Meditation practitioners will awake that they and all creature beings are ones. The delusive mind makes them think that they are separate. Mindfulness in meditation leads to the realization of liberation and enlightenment. Anyone can gain these abilities of mind through meditation. This is the most effective way to gain long-lasting happiness.

Thich Nhat Hanh continued: "Buddha teach pay special attention to observing your breath. Meditate on your body, feelings, mental formations, consciousness, and objects of your consciousness. Look deeply in order to see the process of birth, growth, and fading of every phenomenon, from your own body, emotions, mind, and objects of your mind the happiness liberation brings is true unconditional happiness." Anyone can do and they will understand life is interdependent, timeless, egoless, and emptiness, "all in one and one in all". So that, mindful people will realize what is the most effective way of acting, ones can understand the philosophy of inaction of Lao Tzu, the philosophy of nonviolence of Gandhi, and the philosophy of kindness of Dalai Lama. These simple philosophies are true for all people; it is the root of all other science, education, business, and parenting and governing.

B. Simple mediation practices for busy people:

At home, you can sit cross legs on flat, on a small cushion under the bottom to avoid falling backward or sitting on the coach; where you can have enough quiet and uninterrupted time. Practice daily five to ten minutes in a quiet place. Straighten your body like a feeling of direct force pulls from the head to make upright; then let the body relax in the straight position. Practice some of these exercises of observing. There are people practice meditation for the first time, a lot of thoughts jump out and disappear. It is normal because this is the normal function of the mind. Do not worry, just identifying and naming the thoughts of past, future, positive, negative, nonsense, selfish. After recognizing and naming, thought cannot be self-sustaining, thoughts only sustain when we let ourselves breed and chase the thoughts. Just recognize and name the thoughts then come back to the observing. Practice each of these exercises from five to ten minutes. Whenever you want to stay focus, you can practice observing one of the following exercises.

Exercise one: Observe the relaxation of the whole body.

Stop the thinking process; observing the comfort, relaxation, and lightness of the body. Just breathing in and breathing out with the observing. Practice for at least three to five minutes.

Exercise two: Observe the breath.

Observe the breath in and out, inhalation and exhalation through the noses. Just recognize and observe the breath, do not try to control or adjust the breath. Observing, watching the breath, sensing the path of the breath. Feel the moving of the chest and abdomen when taking a breath. Practice for at least three to five minutes.

Exercise three: Count the breath during meditating

With the position of sitting for meditation, breathe in count one, breathe out count one; next breath, breathe in count two, breathe out count two. Then breathe in count three, breathe out count three. Do count less than five and do not count more than ten. When count to ten, we can count back from one. Practice for at least three to five minutes.

Exercise four: observe the lower abdomen

Observe the lower abdomen when breathing. Breathe in with the observation of moving of the lower abdomen and exhale the observation of moving lower abdomen. Watching the rising and falling of the lower abdomen. Practice for at least three to five minutes.

Exercise five: Observe the lower body in meditating

Observe the lower body when breathing. From the chest down, observe and sense the sensations of the hands, feet, and abdomen. Just observe the parts of the body; just realize the sensation of that lower part. Observe them as empty space

104

cavity moving with the breath. We can feel joy with a sense of lightness and empty. Practice for at least three to five minutes.

If when you observe the body, thoughts appear, this is the normal function of the mind. Just realize the thoughts, do not follow thoughts. Come back to observe the breath. There are people practice meditation for t the, a lot of thinking jump out because of normal function of mind, do not worry, just identify and name the thought like past, future, positive, negative, nonsense, selfish. After naming, thinking cannot be self-sustaining. Just recognize and name the thoughts, then come back to observe the body and the breath. This is the characteristic of mind. Understanding the mind, we can control the power of the mind.

In this practicing of you can practice some of the following breathing techniques, each kind of breath you can do for several minutes. These breathing help you bring joy, happiness, and lightness for yourself, to some extent, it can help to heal your wounds, illnesses.

1. Breath in slowly and breath out with the feeling of happiness, just observing the breathing and feeling, do not try to control them.

2. Breath in slowly and breath out with smiling, just observing, do not try to control them.

3. Breath in with the feeling of lightness, the breath out with the feeling of coolness; just observe the breathing, and feeling of lightness and coolness.

4. Breath in with the feeling of warmness to the whole body, breath out with the feeling of warmness to the whole body, just observes the breath and feeling of warmness.

5. Breath with the feeling of gratitude, breath out with the feeling of joyfulness.

6. Breath in with the feeling of warmness in the body, breath out with the feeling of emptiness in the body.

7. Breath in with the feeling of joy, breath out feels lightness from letting go.

Exercise six: identify the thoughts that appear from the top of the head

It seems like there is a small brain at the top of the head to observe the thoughts appear in the head during meditating. Sitting in meditating position, just observe the thought appear in the head. Identifying and naming thoughts. Just identify, do not follow thoughts. Thoughts will appear and disappear constantly and out of our control. There are some people doing this exercise have a thousand thoughts in just ten minutes of meditating. With the time of practicing, the mind will reduce the habit of jumping around with thinking, and you will know the way to cut off thoughts, over time the mind will calm down. People practice meditation can gain the power of concentration.

> It is the mark of an educated mind to be able to entertain a thought without accepting it. **Aristotle**

Understanding gained by meditation, people can realize that we are wrong when totally believing, clinging to the old thought and protecting the old assumption. Clinging and attaching to previous emotions and assumptions is like covering the eyes with gray clouds. We consciously do not realize that our attachment to constantly changing things cause misery ourselves. With attachment to the previous assumption, we are blind to real facts, and good opinions; moreover, we anger to good but different opinions. Anger is another gray cloud covers our eyes. Many gray clouds of attachment and anger compound day by day into a thick black cloud. Because of attachment and anger, we ourselves make us like blind unconsciously. Looking back at our experiences, we will realize a lot of smart people became blind to the obvious truth when they were angry; their perceptions about facts have distorted. Detachment with any assumptions and detachment with any emotions are some of the ways that great scientists,

106

entrepreneurs, politicians, and people use to do to get the real fact, real knowledge from experiments and events.

By practicing meditation, we can get a better understanding of our mind and our ignorance. We realize the problems we have are not the real problems, they the products of our expectation, our anger, and our ignorance. Understanding makes us more open to different opinions and ideas. We have to remove all assumptions before coming to the situation, we have to listen more, and create open conversations to get understanding. We need to contemplate to create the blueprint of our life first before taking massive actions. We need to find out our talents, strengths, love, and missions. With vivid vision, big goals, principles, values, compassion, serving heart, and persistence, individuals and organizations can achieve far more success than the ones without; these are not only the guiding stars but also the effective tools to direct our mind. Vision, goals, principles, values, compassion are the constants in the changing life; great men always remain constant to these. These are the effective tools for us to win over the self, the ego.

> "Things that I felt absolutely sure of but a few years ago, I do not believe now. This thought makes me see more clearly how foolish it would be to expect all men to agree with me."
>
> "It doesn't matter which side of the fence you get off on sometimes. What matters most is getting off."
>
> **Jim Rohn**

Practice meditation daily in a quiet place. When feelings of anger or negative emotions invade our mind, observe the thoughts and emotions from the top of your head to get a better understanding. Understanding will create compassion and love.

C. Mindfulness prevents us from making mistakes

Daniel Goleman cited a story in a rough neighborhood of New York City where there is a high rate of crimes: violence, robbery, murder. Most students have concentration problems and have witnessed or had relatives killed. Before class, students practiced an exercise of observing the movement of an object placed on the abdomen near the navel for five to ten minutes; this is one of the exercises of breathing in meditation. That daily ritual keeps the class environment calm and constructive and is empowering the children with self-control strategies early on. The class was fun, effective and little aggressive actions during the day. Researchers found that if teachers cut this exercise before class; the class was much more disordered and chaotic, and students were more irritated and aggressive. The scientific research evidence on the benefits of meditation is already compelling, and there are major studies underway.

We are usually anxious before an important interview or test; most of the time, the anxiety is out of controlled. We experience the symptoms of stress; which are the effects of overload stress hormones. Most symptoms of stress that we can find in many patients. Even though, these symptoms may be worse if we still stimulate the mind with the thoughts or images of pain and failure from that event. The negative imagination can create far more fear and anxiety; we may think that we might fail, might make mistakes and might not do well. These thoughts in mind make us more afraid of a real event. The stress symptoms are obvious in the individuals who usually act according to emotion and irrational thinking. The thought itself makes us fall from anxiety to stress with symptoms of sweating, shaking, short breath, forgetting, pale, overreacting and high blood pressure. I see many senior healthy people come to a clinic to get the certification of health to go abroad to visit relatives; the results are good except the blood pressure is higher than the one they check at home. With little relaxation, some of them get high blood pressure near to the number they did at home. In practice, many physicians may see a lot of people have blood pressure rise when they see physicians in the white coat. Many patients are so afraid of injection that when they see a physician in white coat come only to check the blood pressure; most of the time the result may be higher than the patients do by themselves. This is proof that the unconscious mind controls us only with the imagination of the mind. The arousing of the mind can be calm down if we take the right understanding of the situation. In worse cases, if we breed the mind with lots of negative thoughts, the unconscious becoming stronger than the conscious mind. we may fall to extreme stress with a lot of wild actions, which can cause a lot of hurting and misery. When we are anxious, the good advice is to stop thinking, stop chasing the thoughts of past and future by direct the mind back to the body, back the mind to the present. Just by watching the breath, take control to make a deep breath, feel the breath, the sensation in the body, or just by counting the breath; these exercises direct the mind back to the body and cut the unwanted thoughts and make us calmer and less fear than before. When taking control of the mind, we focus the mind to present, we may direct the mind to focus on positive sides and positive figures of the event. Consciously looking to positive sides can make us confident to deal actively with the coming events. Our actions in a calm mind are more conscious and rational than the actions in stress.

Tragedy in the film starts with the knots: a character with power just only sees a small part of the unwanted action from another character, or he just gets distorted information; which he hates so much that he gets angry from perceiving. He makes series of mistakes like: without seeking more information to get the right understanding of the actions, without paying attention to the new emotions, skip reading the context, ignoring all opportunity to learn more about situations and stop digging to the purpose of the action. He hurries to draw out the wrong conclusion. Then he firmly clings to his conclusion and starts to make a series of following behaviors, which are supported by the conclusion. He creates the worst scenario of misunderstanding. These wrong actions cause terrible misery for good character because of misunderstanding. It is even worse than the individuals blindly immersed in bad and evil actions that cause injustice to good characters. During the film, these knots gradually dismantled.

Unfortunately, these tragedies appear all over the world, in countries and in families, because of the ignorance, we unconsciously create a lot of mistakes; the ignorant actions create extreme misery to our beloved people who are totally needed our love and support. Read stories in the newspaper or media we can see these kinds of tragedies in life. There are many successful people talked about the tragedies they got when they were young; fortunately, they bounce back better and get success in life. Oprah Winfrey, Tony Robbins, Steve Job are some of them.

In fact, our ignorance is unlimited; people have killed or created tragedies for many great men in history. Some of the western great men are Christ, Socrates, Galileo Galilei, and Abraham Lincoln. We cannot list all the misery of great caused by people's ignorance.

Unfortunately, ignorance is still in us, and billion other people. If we are not awake to train ourselves to become enlightened, we may create hundreds of ignorant behaviors each day, we may create suffering for relatives, ourselves and all other creatures. Nowadays, most of the wars, the act of terrorism, crimes, mental diseases, health problems, problems in family, schools, and society caused by the desire, anger, and ignorance of the people. Most of the victims and related people have ever experienced the stress symptoms, which listed in table three: the most symptoms of stress that we can find in many patients. Such a terrible, the actions caused misery for people are wearing noble masks of love, justice, peace, development, and sacrifice. Human beings are still be governed by the devil of ignorance. The masks not only make people feel at ease with the wrong actions and but also dull their gut feelings with wrong actions.

We need to practice more to gain wisdom and enlightenment. It is the best way we can do to help our beloved who are suffering. Outside intervention can only make people feel at ease with disease; it cannot eliminate the stress still arousing inside the victims. With enlightenment and wisdom, we can free ourselves and other people from the chains of ignorance.

D. People may be lead to crazy emotion if they lack mindfulness

The stories about the crazy state we can hear a lot from media like someone told that they did not understand what was wrong with them at the time of taking evil actions. They do not know why they do that crime, the action that they never thought of when they are in the normal state of mind. It is like there is a devil drove them to take crazy actions like beatings, stabbing, killing, and creating extreme hurt for others unconsciously.

Right understanding, they are just victims of uncontrolled peak emotions. They are so clingy to the expectation that they believe is true. The expectations were unsatisfied, they became angry. Stimulation of angry emotions made them uncomfortable with some signs. Combine with the chaotic environment, chaotic situation, or the chasing. The crowd, loud voice, loud music, shouting and chasing speed up the pulsating heartbeat, make emotion excited. Accumulation of time and many other unwanted things, their anger reached the peak of emotion. People will lose control of conscious mind when the emotion caused by unconscious my reach to peak. Most of the symptoms in the table two are so vigorous that we can easily realize like the heart rate is very high, the talking same as screaming, the hands are shaking, the pale skin, red face, stiff muscle. The conscious mind loses control of normal behaviors. The emotional brain completely dominates the whole body; on the other hand, the thinking brain is useless. It is like the animals in the extremely dangerous situation; there is no need for thinking, no need for other function put all the resources for fight and flight, put all resources for the irrational behaviors without paying attention for the damaging results. They act in extreme stress unconsciously like crazy men. The actions, at the normal state of mind they never ever think of, are taking.

Sadly, the fact is many parents become crazy with the unwanted actions of their small child. I cannot bear in the mind with the deep wounds, which are bearing by the fragile child trembling with crucial punishments by their crazy but loving parents. The stress distorts all perception from the facts, the distortion creating a more and more vicious circle of hurting.

Family tragedy happens when people fail to read emotional signals, fail to listen to nonverbal signals of themselves and other members. Not understanding or misunderstanding can create anger because they do not get the things they want. So that from small conflicts they do not handle well, they fall to anger, blindly blaming, insulting and shouting each other. They start to ignore the positive evidence, deny the explanation and refuse to cooperate to get understanding. They refuse all pieces of evidence contradicted with their conclusion; on the other hand, their unconscious mind works very efficiently in the situation of strong opinions and high emotions, the unconscious mind starts to scan unwanted things. So that small un-seemingly insignificant things now become the important things in conflict as long as it supports their conclusion, even the mind also call on the previous experiences to support their wrong conclusions. This is the reason for the advice that we should not reason with angry men. Their mind sees small un-seemingly insignificant things as seriously threatening. With distorted information, the calculation of cost and benefit of each decision become wrong and useless. They do not read their emotions and the emotions of the opposite person. The stress of conflicts so high that parents dare to make evil actions with the beloved child, which are not be done when they are in a normal state. Surfing the internet, newspaper, and magazines we see thousands of news of these tragedies and

112

bad actions happen each day. The tragedy has the pattern, if we know it, we can prevent it. In medical, these tragedies created many terms of diseases.

From infants to adolescents or even adults are the victims of ignorant conflicts. Stress, lack of connection and lack of love and the ability of the individual are the ingredients make the quality of people living. If we make a test of the symptoms in table two the most symptoms of stress that we can find in many patients with the patients and people around the patients, we will get outstanding evidence of these causes.

Who let the emotions control so many times; they have been conditioned to the habit of responding in an irrational way. They always meet or create problem unconsciously with other people. Practicing meditation, reducing desires, anger, and ignorance, and forming the seven habits of highly effective people from Stephen Covey can help us not committing the wrong actions.

E. Mindful reading to emotional management

Read environment, read emotion, read the context, read gestures, read linguistic and non-verbal signs, and live in mindfulness. Read what you see, read what you hear, read what you feel. Be aware of the signs of emotion, emotions expressed through non-verbal signals. Some of the best ways are mute the TV, read the actor's feelings for at least ten minutes a day, start analysis scenario, realize the track of emotional development in actors. In the midst of the crowds, parks, or meetings, practice to read the emotions of people around, start with guessing and then finding the clues to sharpen your mind.

Always live in awareness to observe the body, feelings, perceptions, mental formations, and consciousness. Take quiet time to contemplate about the major things in your life. Spend time on major things, awake to do not spend major time on minor things.

ALL IN ONE, ONE IN ALL:

Dear Neurologist, psychiatrist, sociologist, gastroenterologist, urologist, educators, sleep therapists, cardiologist, language therapists, educators, trainers, physiotherapists, and teachers: there is no separation in the health of heart, stomach, muscle, cognitive thinking, sleeping, hormone system: all are interdependent and under the state of mind.

Remember when working with the mind: irrational mind, the giant brain evolved for millions of years, illogical mind and Placebo effects, Neuro-plasticity, Mirror neurons, self-affirmation, self-talk, nocebo effects, T1/2 of all substances, taboos, rituals, religious belief, compound effects, conditioned responses, flexible adaptability, illusive mind, self-healing or self-destroying, irrational thinking, Subliminal message, Marketing of luxury brand, and Hysteria: what do we feed the mind of beings every day? And what if all of these lead to negativity or positivity? Maybe Outliers or Failures!

Thank for reading, I hope that we can be awakened by our beloved people together we can do more!

References:

1. A Level Biology. (n.d.). Factors Affecting Enzyme Activity. Retrieved July 17, 2019, from https://alevelbiology.co.uk/notes/factors-affecting-enzyme-activity/

2. Alina Wo., Bartosz W., Gerard D., Celestyna Mila-K., and Andrzej R. (2007, February 16). The effect of whole-body cryostimulation on lysosomal enzyme activity in kayakers during training. Authors. Authors and affiliations. Original Article. First Online: 16 February 2007. Retrieved July 17, 2019, from https://link.springer.com/article/10.1007/s00421-007-0404-0.

3. Andrea Kurz, MD; Daniel I. Sessler, MD; Richard Christensen, BA; Martha Dechert, BA. (n.d.). Heat Balance and Distribution during the Core-Temperature Plateau in Anesthetized Humans. Retrieved July 17, 2019, fromhttps://anesthesiology.pubs.asahq.org/article.aspx?articleid=2029234

4. Article Navigation. Influence of Dietary Lipid on Lipogenic Enzyme Activities in Coho Salmon, Oncorhynchus kisutch . (Walbaum). Huangsheng Lin Dale R. Romsos Peter I. Tack Gilbert A... Retrieved July 17, 2019, from https://academic.oup.com/jn/article-abstract/107/5/846/4769083

5. Axelrod YK, et al. Crit Care Clin. (2006). Temperature management in acute neurologic disorders. Review article. Department of Neurology. Retrieved July 17, 2019, from https://www.ncbi.nlm.nih.gov/m/pubmed/17239754/?i=6&from=/24365362/related

6. Baking Soda Cancer Studies and pH Medicine Published on May 2, 2012. Reference link https://drsircus.com/cancer/cancer-studies-ph-medicine/

7. Baking Soda Dos and Don'ts. Retrieved July 17, 2019, from https://www.webmd.com/a-to-z-guides/baking-soda-do-dont#1

8. Benefits and Risks of Drinking Baking Soda in Water! . (2011, June 13). Retrieved July 17, 2019, from http://doudyeissa.blogspot.com.es/2011/06/benefits-and-risks-of-drinking-baking.html

9. Boldt. (2018, April 30). 33 Surprising Baking Soda Uses & Remedies. Retrieved July 17, 2019, from https://draxe.com/nutrition/article/baking-soda-uses/

10. Catabolism. (n.d.). In Wikipedia. Retrieved July 17, 2019, from https://en.wikipedia.org/wiki/Catabolism

11. Cell_biology. (n.d.). In Wikipedia. Retrieved July 17, 2019, from https://en.wikipedia.org/wiki/Cell_biology

12. Coenzyme Q10. (n.d.). In Wikipedia. Retrieved July 17, 2019, from https://en.m.wikipedia.org/wiki/Coenzyme_Q10

13. Colleen Huber. (n.d.). Does the Baking Soda Cancer Treatment aka . (Sodium Bicarbonate) Work? Retrieved July 17, 2019, from https://natureworksbest.com/dr-tullio-simoncini-sodium-bicarbonate-cancer-treatment/

14. Corinne O'. Osborn. (2017, December 4). Can I Use Baking Soda to Treat Cancer? Retrieved July 17, 2019, from https://www.healthline.com/health/cancer/baking-soda

15. Could baking soda improve cancer treatment? Published Thursday 31 May 2018. Reference link https://www.medicalnewstoday.com/articles/321970.php

16. Cuyamaca College: Biology 230 Human Anatomy

17. David Jockers. (2016, September 23). Baking Soda: Cancer Treatment Uses for Prevention and Testing. Retrieved July 17, 2019, from https://thetruthaboutcancer.com/baking-soda-uses-cancer/

18. Dimitra K., Ilias V. K., Achilleas M., Sofia K., Alexandra G., and Michael I. K. (2015, January 30). Fever-Range Hyperthermia vs. Hypothermia Effect on Cancer Cell Viability, Proliferation and HSP90 Expression. Retrieved July 17, 2019, from https://www.ncbi.nlm.nih.gov/pmc/articles/PMC4312095/

19. Dr Sircus. (2012, May 2). Baking Soda Cancer Studies and pH Medicine. Retrieved July 17, 2019, from http://drsircus.com/medicine/sodium-bicarbonate-baking-soda/cancer-studies-ph-medicine

20. Effect of long-term cold exposure on antioxidant enzyme activities in a small mammal. Retrieved July 17, 2019, from https://www.sciencedirect.com/science/article/pii/S089158490000263X

21. Effect of temperature on enzyme activity. Retrieved July 17, 2019, from http://academic.brooklyn.cuny.edu/biology/bio4fv/page/enz_act.htm

22. Ekofi Research. (2018, July 12). There is an enzyme that makes a reaction that normally takes 78 million years occur in 18 milliseconds. Retrieved July 17, 2019, from

https://nitro.ekofi.science/this-enzyme-makes-a-reaction-that-normally-takes-78-million-years-occur-in-18-milliseconds/

23. Elevation Of Body Temperature In Disease. Retrieved July 17, 2019, from https://nyaspubs.onlinelibrary.wiley.com/doi/abs/10.1111/j.1749-6632.1964.tb13681.x

24. Enzyme Function Dependent On Temperature. Retrieved July 17, 2019, from https://www.wilsonssyndrome.com/ebook/body-function-dependent-on-body-temperature/enzyme-function-dependent-on-temperature/

25. Enzyme. (n.d.). In Wikipedia. Retrieved July 17, 2019, from https://en.wikipedia.org/wiki/Enzyme

26. Enzymes. (n.d.). In Wikipedia. Retrieved July 17, 2019, from https://www.rsc.org/Education/Teachers/Resources/cfb/enzymes.htm

27. Eva V. Osilla; Sandeep Sharma. (2019, March 16). Physiology, Temperature Regulation. Retrieved July 17, 2019, from https://www.ncbi.nlm.nih.gov/books/NBK507838/

28. Glucose . (n.d.). Retrieved July 17, 2019, from https://vi.m.wikipedia.org/wiki/Glucose

29. Gomez CR. Handb Clin Neurol. (2014).Disorders of body temperature. Retrieved July 17, 2019, from https://www.ncbi.nlm.nih.gov/m/pubmed/24365362/

30. Hector Corsi. (2012,APR 25). Baking soda might have potential against cancer. Retrieved July 17, 2019, from http://digitaljournal.com/article/323645

31. Hiromi Shinya. The Enzyme Factor. Source Amazon.com

32. Home remedies for life. (2018, April 22). Baking Soda: 12 Benefits, Properties, Dosage And Side Effects. Retrieved July 17, 2019, from https://homeremediesforlife.com/baking-soda-benefits/

33. Hyperglycemia. (n.d.). In Wikipedia. Retrieved July 17, 2019, fromhttps://en.m.wikipedia.org/wiki/Hyperglycemia

34. Hyperthermia in Cancer Treatment - . Retrieved July 17, 2019, from https://www.cancer.gov/about-cancer/treatment/types/surgery/hyperthermia-fact-sheet

35. Hyperthermia to Treat Cancer. Retrieved July 17, 2019, from https://amp.cancer.org/treatment/treatments-and-side-effects/treatment-types/hyperthermia.html

36. HYPERTHERMIA TREATMENT. Retrieved July 17, 2019, from https://www.texasoncology.com/cancer-blood-disorders/cancer-facts/hyperthermia-treatment

37. Hyperthermia: Role and Risk Factor for Cancer Treatment. Retrieved July 17, 2019, from https://www.sciencedirect.com/science/article/pii/S2078152016 300724

38. Hypertriglyceridemia. (n.d.). In Wikipedia. Retrieved July 17, 2019, from https://en.wikipedia.org/wiki/Hypertriglyceridemia

39. Hypoglycemia. (n.d.). In Wikipedia. Retrieved July 17, 2019, from https://en.m.wikipedia.org/wiki/Hypoglycemia

40. Hypotension. (n.d.). In Wikipedia. Retrieved July 17, 2019, from https://en.m.wikipedia.org/wiki/Hypotension

41. Hypotension/Low Blood Pressure: Symptoms, Complications, and Treatment. (n.d.). In Wikipedia. Retrieved July 17, 2019, from https://www.practo.com/health-wiki/hypotension-low-blood-pressure-symptoms-complications-and-treatment/3/article

42. Hypothermia and cancer chemotherapy. Retrieved July 17, 2019, from https://www.ncbi.nlm.nih.gov/m/pubmed/5812564/

43. Hypothermia -Chapter 76 - Author links open overlay panelPeter J.FagenholzMDEdward A.BittnerMD, PhD. Available online 14 September 2012.

44. Hypothermia -Shelley Wells Collins. Retrieved July 17, 2019, from https://www.cancertherapyadvisor.com/home/decision-support-in-medicine/hospital-medicine/hypothermia/

45. Hypothermia. (n.d.). In Wikipedia. Retrieved July 17, 2019, from https://en.m.wikipedia.org/wiki/Hypothermia

46. Hypothermia. , in Complications in Anesthesia . (Second Edition), 2007

47. Hypothermia. Peter J. Fagenholz MD, Edward A. Bittner MD, PhD, in Critical Care Secrets . (Fifth Edition).

48. Introduction to Enzymes. Retrieved July 17, 2019, from http://www.worthington-biochem.com/introbiochem/tempEffects.html

49. Ivayla I Ge., Brian C., Tasaduq F., Waleed J. (3019, April). Normal Body Temperature: Systematic Review. Retrieved July 17, 2019, from https://academic.oup.com/ofid/article/6/4/ofz032/5435701

50. Jessie A. Key. (n.d.). Factors that Affect the Rate of Reactions. Retrieved July 17, 2019, from https://opentextbc.ca/introductorychemistry/chapter/factors-that-affect-the-rate-of-reactions-2/

51. Joseph West. (n.d.). Why Does Heating Interfere With the Activity of an Enzyme? Retrieved July 17, 2019, from https://sciencing.com/why-does-heating-interfere-with-the-activity-of-an-enzyme-12730636.html

52. Khalid S.., Rafat A. S. (2017, August 281). Papaya black seeds have beneficial anticancer effects on PC-3 prostate cancer cells. Retrieved July 17, 2019, from https://jcmtjournal.com/article/view/2224

53. Kinetics: Determination of an Enzymes Activity – Relevance. Retrieved July 17, 2019, from https://www.chem.fsu.edu/chemlab/bch4053l/enzymes/activity/index.html

54. Lloyd Jenkins. (2015, June 29) . Fight Disease and Fatigue with Lemon Juice and Baking Soda. Retrieved July 17, 2019, from https://budwigcenter.com/fight-disease-and-fatigue-with-lemon-juice-and-baking-soda/

55. Matthew Lee. (2018, December 12), Metabolizing Proteins Vs. Fats. Retrieved July 17, 2019, from https://healthyeating.sfgate.com/metabolizing-proteins-vs-fats-3453.html

56. Mayer FQ, et al. Artif Organs. (2010). Effects of cryopreservation and hypothermic storage on cell viability and enzyme activity in recombinant encapsulated cells overexpressing alpha-L-iduronidase. Retrieved July 17, 2019, from https://www.ncbi.nlm.nih.gov/m/pubmed/20633158/

57. Mdhealth. (n.d.). How to Drink Baking Soda for Optimal Results. Retrieved July 17, 2019, from http://www.md-health.com/Drinking-Baking-Soda.html

58. Melinda Ratini. (2018, March 13). Unexplained Nerve Pain. Retrieved July 17, 2019, from https://www.webmd.com/pain-management/unexplained-nerve-pain-the-mystery-of-neuropathic-pain#1

59. Melinda Ratini. (2018, March 16). Nerve Pain and Nerve Damage. Retrieved July 17, 2019, from

https://www.webmd.com/brain/nerve-pain-and-nerve-damage-symptoms-and-causes#1

60. Metabolic_syndrome. (n.d.). In Wikipedia. Retrieved July 17, 2019, from https://en.wikipedia.org/wiki/Metabolic_syndrome

61. Metabolism. (n.d.). In Wikipedia. Retrieved July 17, 2019, from https://en.m.wikipedia.org/wiki/Metabolism

62. Molecular mechanisms of temperature compensation in poikilotherms.. J R Hazel, and C L Prosser. Retrieved July 17, 2019, from https://www.physiology.org/doi/abs/10.1152/physrev.1974.54.3.620

63. Neuropathic pain. (n.d.). In Wikipedia. Retrieved July 17, 2019, from https://en.wikipedia.org/wiki/Neuropathic_pain

64. Ngoc D. Do. (2016, November 5). Đột phá nghiên cứu mới cho biết Làm thế nào để đảo ngược khỏi bệnh tiểu đường trong 3 tuần. Retrieved July 17, 2019, from http://khicongydaododucngoc.blogspot.com/2016/11/ot-pha-nghien-cuu-moi-cho-biet-lam-nao.html

65. Ngoc D. Do. (2016, November 5). Nhịp tim liên quan đến : Khí . (tâm thu), Huyết . (tâm trương), đường. Retrieved July 17, 2019, from http://khicongydaododucngoc.blogspot.com/2016/11/nhip-tim-lien-quan-en-khi-tam-thu-huyet_5.html

66. Ngoc D. Do. (n.d.) Chua Dau Lung : Khi Cong Tinh Do , Thay Do Duc Ngoc EIAB Germany 2014. Retrieved July 17, 2019, from http://khicongydaododucngoc.blogspot.com/

67. Peter Janiszewski(December 2, 2015). How long can humans survive without food or water? Retrieved July 17, 2019, from https://medicalxpress.com/news/2015-12-humans-survive-food.html

68. Protease inhibitor . (biology). (n.d.). In Wikipedia. Retrieved July 17, 2019, from https://en.m.wikipedia.org/wiki/Protease_inhibitor_. (biology)

69. Protein catabolism. (n.d.). In Wikipedia. Retrieved July 17, 2019, from https://en.wikipedia.org/wiki/Protein_catabolism

70. Protein–energy malnutrition. (n.d.). In Wikipedia. Retrieved July 17, 2019, from

https://en.wikipedia.org/wiki/Protein%E2%80%93energy_malnu trition

71. Proteins and Temperature. Annual Review of Physiology. Vol. 57:43-68 . (Volume publication date March 1995). Retrieved July 17, 2019, from https://doi.org/10.1146/annurev.ph.57.030195.000355. Retrieved July 17, 2019, from https://www.annualreviews.org/doi/pdf/10.1146/annurev.ph.57 .030195.000355

72. Sam Blanchard. (2018, May 31). Drinking baking soda could help cure cancer: Kitchen ingredient makes hard-to-reach tumour cells easier to target with drugs, study finds. Retrieved July 17, 2019, from https://www.dailymail.co.uk/health/article-5791377/Baking-soda-make-hard-reach-tumour-cells-easier-target-chemotherapy.html

73. Sandi Busch. (n.d.). How Quickly Does Protein Metabolize? Retrieved July 17, 2019, from https://www.livestrong.com/article/550839-how-quickly-does-protein-metabolize/

74. Sci –News. (2018, June 6). Baking Soda Could Improve Cancer Therapy. Retrieved July 17, 2019, from http://www.sci-news.com/medicine/baking-soda-cancer-therapy-06071.html

75. Science Experiments Demonstrating How Temperature Affects Enzyme Activity. Retrieved July 17, 2019, from https://education.seattlepi.com/science-experiments-demonstrating-temperature-affects-enzyme-activity-6633.html.

76. Secondary metabolite. (n.d.). In Wikipedia. Retrieved July 17, 2019, from https://en.m.wikipedia.org/wiki/Secondary_metabolite

77. Sickle cell disease. (n.d.). In Wikipedia. Retrieved July 17, 2019, from https://en.wikipedia.org/wiki/Sickle_cell_disease

78. Sindhu R., Binod P., Sabeela B. U., Amith A., Anil K. M.,Aravind M., Sharrel R., and Ashok P. (2018, Mar). Applications of Microbial Enzymes in Food Industry. Retrieved July 17, 2019, from https://www.ncbi.nlm.nih.gov/pmc/articles/PMC5956270/

79. The Effects of Temperature on Enzyme Activity and Biology. Retrieved July 17, 2019, from https://sciencing.com/effects-temperature-enzyme-activity-biology-6049.html

80. Traditional Asian medicine. Retrieved July 17, 2019, from https://en.m.wikipedia.org/wiki/Traditional_Asian_medicine
81. Traditional Chinese medicine. (n.d.). In Wikipedia. Retrieved July 17, 2019, from https://en.m.wikipedia.org/wiki/Traditional_Chinese_medicine
82. Traditional medicine. (n.d.). Retrieved July 17, 2019, from https://en.m.wikipedia.org/wiki/Traditional_medicine
83. Traditional Vietnamese medicine. Retrieved July 17, 2019, from https://en.m.wikipedia.org/wiki/Traditional_Vietnamese_medicine
84. Van D. Dao. (2018, February 25). The hidden relation, clues of autism, ADHD and depression which reveals the cause and possible cure. Retrieved July 17, 2019, from http://www.awakenyouwonderfulwe.com/2018/11/the-hidden-relation-clues-of-autism_13.html.
85. Van D. Dao. (2018, March 07). Real cause of human problems: Autism, ADHD, Depression, Suicide and Stress. Retrieved July 17, 2019, from http://www.awakenyouwonderfulwe.com/2018/07/real-cause-of-human-problems-autism.html
86. Van D. Dao. (2019, July 17). Simple meditation and the teaching of Thich Nhat Hanh, Buddha teaching to practice for busy people to calm the mind and cure the disorders. Retrieved July 17, 2019, from http://www.awakenyouwonderfulwe.com/2018/01/simple-mediation-and-teaching-of-thich.html
87. Van D. Dao. (n.d) New view of diseases that helps healing most chronic diseases, chronic problems. Retrieved July 17, 2019, from http://www.awakenyouwonderfulwe.com/2018/01/new-view-of-diseases-that-helps-healing.html.
88. Van D. Dao. (n.d.). AWAKEN YOU WONDERFUL WE: The secret of one-page table reveal all the real causes of all phenomena and problems: Most phenomena, physical problems, mental problems, social problems and how to solve them: Ability, Autoimmune diseases, Belief system... Retrieved July 17, 2019, from https://www.amazon.com/Awaken-you-wonderful-phenomena-problems/dp/1549843524
89. Van D. Dao. (October, 2019). The cause and possible cure for cancer and chronic diseases from applying Papaya leaf juice,

baking soda, aspirin, sugar, temperature, Vietnamese Qi Gong breathing, exercise, metabolism, and traditional medicine.

90. Van D. Duy. (2019, August). Ứng dụng thiền và khí công theo nguyên lý YHCT giúp tăng cường sức khỏe, phòng và chữa bệnh. Retrieved August 27, 2019, from https://edumall.vn/course/ung-dung-thien-va-khi-cong-theo-nguyen-ly-yhct-giup-tang-cuong-suc-khoe-phong-va-chua-benh.html

91. Van Duy Dao. "The Relation between Smoking, Breathing, Glycemia and the Rate of the Metabolism that Reveals the Effective Way of Controlling Body Weight and Glycemia". Acta Scientific Neurology 2.9 . (2019): 15-20.

92. Vitamin A. (n.d.). In Wikipedia. Retrieved July 17, 2019, from https://en.m.wikipedia.org/wiki/Vitamin_A

93. Vitamin C. (n.d.). In Wikipedia. Retrieved July 17, 2019, from https://en.m.wikipedia.org/wiki/Vitamin_C

94. Vitamin E. (n.d.). In Wikipedia. Retrieved July 17, 2019, from https://en.m.wikipedia.org/wiki/Vitamin_E

95. Webster Kehr. (2019, June 5). Vitamin c and baking soda cancer treatment including cancers of the digestive tract. Reference link https://www.cancertutor.com/vitc_bsoda/

96. William P. C., San P. Rd., and Jacksonville,. (2016, January 5). Thermoregulatory disorders and illness related to heat and cold stress. Retrieved July 17, 2019, from https://www.sciencedirect.com/science/article/pii/S1566070216300017

97. Worthington. (n.d.) Introduction to Enzymes. Retrieved July 17, 2019, from http://www.worthington-biochem.com/introbiochem/factors.html

98. Yin and yang. Retrieved July 17, 2019, from https://en.m.wikipedia.org/wiki/Yin_and_yang

99. References the cause and possible cure:

100. 15 Best Health Benefits of Eating Papaya. (n.d.). In Wikipedia. Retrieved July 17, 2019, from https://www.gyanunlimited.com/health/papaya-benefits-and-nutritional-facts-of-papaya/5960/

101. A Level Biology. (n.d.). Factors Affecting Enzyme Activity. Retrieved July 17, 2019, from

https://alevelbiology.co.uk/notes/factors-affecting-enzyme-activity/

102. AIDS. (n.d.). In Wikipedia. Retrieved July 17, 2019, from https://en.wikipedia.org/wiki/HIV/AIDS

103. Back_pain. (n.d.). In Wikipedia. Retrieved July 17, 2019, from https://en.wikipedia.org/wiki/Back_pain

104. Berenice Hudson. (2015). EPIDEMIOLOGY. General Prevalence of Acute Pain Lifetime prevalence in general population: – Approaches 100% for acute pain leading to use of analgesics. Retrieved July 17, 2019, from https://slideplayer.com/slide/4886109/

105. Blood sugar level. (n.d.). In Wikipedia. Retrieved July 17, 2019, from https://en.m.wikipedia.org/wiki/Blood_sugar_level

106. Blood sugar regulation. (n.d.). In Wikipedia. Retrieved July 17, 2019, from https://en.m.wikipedia.org/wiki/Blood_sugar_regulation

107. Breast_cancer. (n.d.). In Wikipedia. Retrieved July 17, 2019, from https://en.wikipedia.org/wiki/Breast_cancer

108. Canceractive. (2018, September 5). Acid Bodies increase cancer risk and metastases. Retrieved July 17, 2019, from http://www.canceractive.com/cancer-active-page-link.aspx?n=1025

109. Carol DerSarkissian. (2018, February 28). Home Remedies for Nerve Pain. Retrieved July 17, 2019, from https://www.webmd.com/pain-management/nerve-pain-self-care#1

110. Carol DerSarkissian. (2018, May 3). Nonprescription Treatments for Nerve Pain. Retrieved July 17, 2019, from https://www.webmd.com/pain-management/nonprescription-treatments-nerve-pain#1

111. Carol DerSarkissian. (2018, May 3). Prescription Medications and Treatments for Nerve Pain. Retrieved July 17, 2019, from https://www.webmd.com/pain-management/prescription-medications-treatments-nerve-pain#1

112. Catia G., Michele B., Marco B. T., Matteo C.,Luigi B.,and Laura G.. (2017, March 21). Venom from Cuban Blue Scorpion has tumor activating effect in hepatocellular carcinom. Retrieved July 17, 2019, from https://www.ncbi.nlm.nih.gov/pmc/articles/PMC5359575/

113. Chest_pain. (n.d.). In Wikipedia. Retrieved July 17, 2019, from https://en.wikipedia.org/wiki/Chest_pain

114. Diabetes. (n.d.). In Wikipedia. Retrieved July 17, 2019, from https://en.wikipedia.org/wiki/Diabetes

115. Elizabeth Mendes. (2015, September 24). Aspirin and Cancer Prevention: What the Research Really Shows. Retrieved July 17, 2019, from https://www.cancer.org/latest-news/aspirin-and-cancer-prevention-what-the-research-really-shows.html

116. Enzyme Activity. Last updatedJun 6, 2019. Retrieved July 17, 2019, from https://chem.libretexts.org/Bookshelves/Introductory_Chemistry/Book%3A_The_Basics_of_GOB_Chemistry_. (Ball_et_al.)/18%3A_Amino_Acids%2C_Proteins%2C_and_Enzymes/18.07_Enzyme_Activity

117. Ethan Boldt. (2018, April 30). 33 Surprising Baking Soda Uses & Remedies. Retrieved July 17, 2019, from https://draxe.com/nutrition/article/baking-soda-uses/

118. Fabrizio R., Raffaele D. C., Artur F. (2015, August 18). Orthostatic Hypotension: Epidemiology, Prognosis, and Treatment. Retrieved July 17, 2019, from https://www.sciencedirect.com/science/article/pii/S073510971503939X

119. Fatma Al-Maskari. (2010, July). Lifestyle diseases: An Economic Burden on the Health Services By . Retrieved July 17, 2019, from https://unchronicle.un.org/article/lifestyle-diseases-economic-burden-health-services

120. Fatma Al-Maskari. (2010, July). Lifestyle Diseases: An Economic Burden on the Health Services. Retrieved July 17, 2019, from https://unchronicle.un.org/article/lifestyle-diseases-economic-burden-health-services

121. Fever, fever patterns and diseases called 'fever' – A review. Retrieved July 17, 2019, from https://www.sciencedirect.com/science/article/pii/S1876034111000256

122. Fever. Retrieved July 17, 2019, from https://www.mayoclinic.org/diseases-conditions/fever/symptoms-causes/syc-20352759

123. Fever: The Rules Change After a Cancer Diagnosis. Retrieved July 17, 2019, from

https://www.roswellpark.org/cancertalk/201807/fever-rules-change-after-cancer-diagnosis

124.Final Recommendation Statement. Aspirin Use to Prevent Cardiovascular Disease and Colorectal Cancer: Preventive Medication. (2016, April). Retrieved July 17, 2019, from https://www.uspreventiveservicestaskforce.org/Page/Document /RecommendationStatementFinal/aspirin-to-prevent-cardiovascular-disease-and-cancer

125.Five elements . (Chinese philosophy). Retrieved July 17, 2019, from https://psychology.wikia.org/wiki/Five_elements_. (Chinese_philosophy)

126.Ford, Earl S; Bergmann, Manuela M; Kroger, Janine; Schienkiewitz, Anja; Weikert, Cornelia; Boeing, Heiner. "Healthy Living Is the Best Revenge: Findings From the European Prospective Investigation Into Cancer and Nutrition-Potsdam Study", Arch Intern Med, 169 . (15) . (2009): 1355-1362.

127.Fran Kritz. (2018, Ocotober 22). Lack of Exercise Poses a Greater Health Risk Than Smoking, Diabetes, and Heart Disease - Research tracks "the relationship between extremely high fitness and mortality." Retrieved July 17, 2019, from https://www.everydayhealth.com/heart-health/lack-exercise-poses-greater-health-risk-than-smoking-diabetes-heart-disease/

128.Fran Kritz. (2018, October 22). Lack of Exercise Poses a Greater Health Risk Than Smoking, Diabetes, and Heart Disease. Research tracks "the relationship between extremely high fitness and mortality." Retrieved July 17, 2019, from https://www.everydayhealth.com/heart-health/lack-exercise-poses-greater-health-risk-than-smoking-diabetes-heart-disease/

129.Garry Egger, John Dixon. (2014), Beyond Obesity and Lifestyle: A Review of 21st Century Chronic Disease Determinants. Retrieved July 17, 2019, from https://www.hindawi.com/journals/bmri/2014/731685/

130.Hannah Nichols. (2019, July 4). What are the leading causes of death in the US? Retrieved July 17, 2019, from https://www.medicalnewstoday.com/articles/282929.php

131.Health Risks of an Inactive Lifestyle. Also called: Sedentary Lifestyle, Sitting Disease. Retrieved July 17, 2019, from https://medlineplus.gov/healthrisksofaninactivelifestyle.html

132. HIV. (n.d.). In Wikipedia. Retrieved July 17, 2019, from https://en.wikipedia.org/wiki/HIV

133. Hope S. R., Jeffrey V. (n.d.). Scalp Hypothermia for Preventing Alopecia. During Chemotherapy. A Systematic Review and. Meta-Analysis of Randomized Controlled Trials. Retrieved July 17, 2019, from https://www.clinical-breast-cancer.com/article/S1526-8209. (16)30543-2/pdf

134. How to Massage Your Pressure Points. By Peggy Pletcher, MS, RD, LD, CDE on March 25, 2015 — Written by Healthline Editorial Team. Retrieved July 17, 2019, from https://www.healthline.com/health/pain-relief/how-to-massage-your-pressure-points#1

135. Hypothermia. Peter J. Fagenholz MD, Edward A. Bittner MD, PhD, in Critical Care Secrets . (Fifth Edition),

136. India Times. (2019, March 22). 11 Lifestyle diseases you should take seriously. Retrieved July 17, 2019, from https://timesofindia.indiatimes.com/life-style/health-fitness/health-news/11-lifestyle-diseases-you-should-take-seriously/articleshow/16419598.cms

137. Indran M, Mahmood AA, Kuppusamy UR. Protective effect of Carica papaya L leaf extract against alcohol induced acute gastric damage and blood oxidative stress in rats. West Indian Med J. Sep 2008;57. (4):323-326.

138. International Journal of Hyperthermia. Targeting therapy-resistant cancer stem cells by hyperthermia. Retrieved July 17, 2019, from https://www.tandfonline.com/doi/full/10.1080/02656736.2017.1279757

139. J. R. Beaton and , T. Orme. A NOTE ON THE EFFECTS OF HYPOTHERMIA ON ENZYME ACTIVITIES IN THE RAT. Canadian Journal of Biochemistry and Physiology, 1961, 39. (10): 1649-1652, Retrieved July 17, 2019, from https://www.nrcresearchpress.com/doi/abs/10.1139/o61-179#.XSxytOgzblU

140. Jose-Alberto P., Horacio K. (2017, January 30). Epidemiology, Diagnosis, and Management of Neurogenic Orthostatic Hypotension. Retrieved July 17, 2019, from https://onlinelibrary.wiley.com/doi/full/10.1002/mdc3.12478

141. Juárez-Rojop IE, Díaz-Zagoya JC, Ble-Castillo JL, et al. Hypoglycemic effect of Carica papaya leaves in streptozotocin-induced diabetic rats.BMC Complement Altern Med. 2012 Nov 28;12:236.

142. Julie J. Martin. (n.d.). Hypothermia. Retrieved July 17, 2019, from https://www.cancercarewny.com/content.aspx?chunkiid=99914

143. Kazem R., Connor A. E., , and Stephen M. M. (2015, March 13). The Epidemiology of Blood Pressure and Its Worldwide Management. Retrieved July 17, 2019, from https://www.ahajournals.org/doi/full/10.1161/CIRCRESAHA.116. 304723

144. Khí Công Y Đạo, Thầy Đỗ Đức Ngọc giảng về tầm quan trọng nhất của đường theo đông y . 2015. Retrieved July 17, 2019, from http://khicongydaododucngoc.blogspot.com

145. Kidney failure. (n.d.). https://en.wikipedia.org/wiki/Kidney_failure

146. Kris Gunnars. (2018, July 16). A Low-Carb Meal Plan and Menu to Improve Your Health. Retrieved July 17, 2019, from https://www.healthline.com/nutrition/low-carb-diet-meal-plan-and-menu

147. Laura J. Martin. (2018, July 8). Treating Nerve Pain Caused by Cancer, HIV, and Other Conditions. Retrieved July 17, 2019, from https://www.webmd.com/pain-management/treating-nerve-pain-caused-cancer-hiv

148. Leprosy. (n.d.). In Wikipedia. Retrieved July 17, 2019, from https://en.wikipedia.org/wiki/Leprosy

149. List of traditional Chinese medicines. Retrieved July 17, 2019, from https://en.m.wikipedia.org/wiki/List_of_traditional_Chinese_me dicines

150. Lloyd Jenkins. (2015, June 29) . Fight Disease and Fatigue with Lemon Juice and Baking Soda. Retrieved July 17, 2019, from https://budwigcenter.com/fight-disease-and-fatigue-with-lemon-juice-and-baking-soda/

151. Nguyen TT, Parat MO, Shaw PN, et al. Traditional Aboriginal Preparation Alters the Chemical Profile of Carica papaya Leaves

and Impacts on Cytotoxicity towards Human Squamous Cell Carcinoma.PLoS One. 2016;11. (2):e0147956.

152. Palma J., Kaufmann H. (2017, March 16). Epidemiology, Diagnosis, and Management of Neurogenic Orthostatic Hypotension. Retrieved July 17, 2019, from https://www.ncbi.nlm.nih.gov/pubmed/28713844

153. Parkinson disease. (n.d.). In Wikipedia. Retrieved July 17, 2019, from https://en.wikipedia.org/wiki/Parkinson%27s_disease

154. Peter J. F., Edward A. B. (2013). Hypothermia. Combination TherapyCore Temperature. Retrieved July 17, 2019, from https://www.sciencedirect.com/topics/nursing-and-health-professions/hypothermia

155. Protein metabolism. (n.d.). In Wikipedia. Retrieved July 17, 2019, from https://en.m.wikipedia.org/wiki/Protein_metabolism

156. Quist Christina. (n.d). Hypothermia. Retrieved July 17, 2019, from https://www.cancertherapyadvisor.com/home/decision-support-in-medicine/hospital-medicine/hypothermia-2/

157. Sandeep S., Priyanka T. B. (2019, June 20). Hypotension. Retrieved July 17, 2019, from

158. Suy Than : Khi Cong Tinh Do , Do Duc Ngoc EIAB Germany 2014. Retrieved July 17, 2019, from http://khicongydaododucngoc.blogspot.com/

159. Sy Kraft. (2018, August 17). Everything you need to know about hypothermia. Retrieved July 17, 2019, from https://www.medicalnewstoday.com/articles/182197.php

160. Thầy Đỗ Đức Ngọc: Nói về món ăn, thuốc uống thuộc TÌNH 2017 tại Như Tịnh Thất. Retrieved July 17, 2019, from http://khicongydaododucngoc.blogspot.com/

161. Van D. Dao. (2018, May 3). Life is not paradoxical, life is art. Life is not calculated by autistic robot, life is must felt and created. Retrieved July 17, 2019, from http://www.awakenyouwonderfulwe.com/2018/03/life-is-not-paradoxical-life-is-art.html

162. Van D. Dao. (2018, November 15). Seasonal Stress in America and World kill the most, not cold, heat or flu. Retrieved July 17, 2019, from http://www.awakenyouwonderfulwe.com/2017/09/seasonal-stress-in-america-kill-most.html.

163. Van D. Dao. (2019, Fabruary 16). Are autism, depression, ADHD, talented, mastery, poor learning, stress, seizures, drugs, violence, PTSD born or created? Retrieved July 17, 2019, from http://www.awakenyouwonderfulwe.com/2019/02/are-autism-depression-adhd-talented.html.

164. Altus P, Hickman JW (May 1981). Accidental hypothermia: hypoglycemia or hyperglycemia. West. J. Med. 134 (5): 455–6. PMC 1272797. PMID 7257359.

165. Axelrod, Yekaterina K.; Diringer, Michael N. (May 2008). Temperature management in acute neurologic disorders. Neurologic Clinics. 26 (2): 585–603, xi. doi:10.1016/j.ncl.2008.02.005. PMID 18514828.

166. Better Health Channel. (n.d.). Quitting smoking and managing weight. Retrieved July 17, 2019, from https://www.betterhealth.vic.gov.au/health/healthyliving/smoking-and-weight

167. Blood sugar regulation. https://en.m.wikipedia.org/wiki/Blood_sugar_regulation

168. Booth J (November 1977). A short history of blood pressure measurement. Proceedings of the Royal Society of Medicine. 70 (11): 793–9. PMC 1543468. PMID 341169.

169. Bracker, Mark (2012). The 5-Minute Sports Medicine Consult (2 ed.). Lippincott Williams & Wilkins. p. 320. ISBN 9781451148121. Archived from the original on 2017-09-08.

170. Branch Jr., William T.; Barton, Jason J. S. (February 10, 2011). Approach to the patient with dizziness. UpToDate.

171. Brian Krans. (2013, August 21). Heavy Smokers More Likely to Gain Weight When They Quit. Retrieved July 17, 2019, from https://www.healthline.com/health-news/aging-heavy-smokers-gain-more-weight-082113

172. Brown DJ, Brugger H, Boyd J, Paal P (November 2012). Accidental hypothermia. The New England Journal of Medicine. 367 (20): 1930–8. doi:10.1056/NEJMra1114208. PMC 1944204. PMID 23150960.

173. Camille N. Pagán. (2019, January 16).). How to Avoid Gaining Weight When You Quit Smoking. Retrieved July 17, 2019, from https://www.webmd.com/smoking-cessation/features/quit-without-weight-gain#1

174. CDC - NIOSH Workplace Safety and Health Topic - Cold Stress - Cold Related Illnesses. www.cdc.gov. 2018-06-06. Retrieved 2018-08-01.

175. Lakshmi Santhosh (2018, March 14). The Effects of Temperature on Enzyme Activity and Biology. Retrieved July 17, 2019, from https://sciencing.com/two-ways-inhibit-enzyme-activity-11541.html

176. Cold Stress. Center for Disease Control and Prevention. Archived from the original on 2012-08-11. Marx 2010 p.1862

177. Common Side Effects of Coumadin (Warfarin Sodium) Drug Center – RxList. rxlist.com. Retrieved 17 April 2018.

178. Dealing with Weight Gain. (n.d.). Retrieved July 17, 2019, from https://smokefree.gov/challenges-when-quitting/weight-gain-appetite/dealing-with-weight-gain

179. Dizziness and Vertigo. Merck Manual. 2009.

180. Dizziness at Dorland's Medical Dictionary

181. Dizziness at the US National Library of Medicine Medical Subject Headings (MeSH)

182. eMedicine Specialties > Emergency Medicine > Environmental >Hypothermia Archived 2016-03-05 at the Wayback Machine Author: Jamie Alison Edelstein, MD. Coauthors: James Li, MD; Mark A Silverberg, MD; Wyatt Decker, MD. Updated: Oct 29, 2009

183. Gina Shaw. (2019,January 23). Stopping Weight Gain While Quitting Smoking. Many people who quit smoking gain 10 pounds, but not you. Retrieved July 17, 2019, from https://www.webmd.com/smoking-cessation/features/stopping-weight-gain-while-quitting-smoking#1

184. Glucose. (n.d.). In Wikipedia. Retrieved July 17, 2019, from https://vi.m.wikipedia.org/wiki/Glucose

185. Grim CE, Grim CM (March 2016). Auscultatory BP: still the gold standard. Journal of the American Society of Hypertension. 10 (3): 191–3. doi:10.1016/j.jash.2016.01.004. PMID 26839183.

186. Hanania NA, Zimmerman JL (1999). Accidental hypothermia. Crit Care Clin. 15 (2): 235–49. doi:10.1016/s0749-0704(05)70052-x. PMID 10331126.

187. Hypoglycemia. In Wikipedia. Retrieved July 17, 2019, from https://en.m.wikipedia.org/wiki/hypothermia

188.Hypotension. In Wikipedia. Retrieved July 17, 2019, from https://en.m.wikipedia.org/wiki/Hypotension

189.Hypothermia. In Wikipedia. Retrieved July 17, 2019, from https://en.m.wikipedia.org/wiki/Hypothermia

190.IQOSmag. (n.d.). Quitting smoking is possible, but what do to with increasing weight? How not to gain weight when quitting. Retrieved July 17, 2019, from https://www.iqosmag.com/Quitting-smoking-is-possible-but-what-do-to-with-increasing-weight-How-not-to-gain-weight-when-quitting-A_6446

191.Karakitsos D, Karabinis A (September 2008). Hypothermia therapy after traumatic brain injury in children. N. Engl. J. Med. 359 (11): 1179–80. doi:10.1056/NEJMc081418. PMID 18788094.

192.Karatas, Mehmet (2008). Central vertigo and dizziness: epidemiology, differential diagnosis, and common causes. The Neurologist. 14 (6): 355–64. doi:10.1097/NRL.0b013e31817533a3. ISSN 1074-7931. PMID 19008741.

193.Laupland, Kevin B. (July 2009). Fever in the critically ill medical patient. Critical Care Medicine. 37 (7 Suppl): S273–8. doi:10.1097/CCM.0b013e3181aa6117. PMID 19535958.

194.Linda J. Vorvick. (2018, August 3). Weight gain after quitting smoking: What to do. Retrieved July 17, 2019, from https://medlineplus.gov/ency/patientinstructions/000811.htm

195.Marx J (2006). Rosen's emergency medicine: concepts and clinical practice. Mosby/Elsevier. p. 2239. ISBN 978-0-323-02845-5.

196.Marx J (2010). Rosen's emergency medicine: concepts and clinical practice 7th edition. Philadelphia, PA: Mosby/Elsevier. p. 1870. ISBN 978-0-323-05472-0.

197.McCullough L, Arora S (December 2004). Diagnosis and treatment of hypothermia. Am Fam Physician. 70 (12): 2325–32. PMID 15617296.

198.MedlinePlus. (n.d.). Weight gain after quitting smoking: What to do. Retrieved July 17, 2019, from https://medlineplus.gov/ency/patientinstructions/000811.htm

199.Neuhauser HK, Lempert T (November 2009). Vertigo: epidemiologic aspects (PDF). Semin Neurol. 29 (5): 473–81. doi:10.1055/s-0029-1241043. PMID 19834858.

200.Ngoc D. Duc. (2016, November 5). Đột phá nghiên cứu mới cho biết Làm thế nào để đảo ngược khỏi bệnh tiểu đường trong 3 tuần. Retrieved July 17, 2019, from ttp://khicongydaododucngoc.blogspot.com/2016/11/ot-pha-nghien-cuu-moi-cho-biet-lam-nao.html

201.Ngoc D. Duc. (2016, November 5). Nhịp tim liên quan đến : Khí (tâm thu), Huyết (tâm trương), đường. Retrieved July 17, 2019, from http://khicongydaododucngoc.blogspot.com/2016/11/nhip-tim-lien-quan-en-khi-tam-thu-huyet_5.html

202.Ngoc D. Duc. (n.d.). Nói về món ăn, thuốc uống tại Như Tịnh Thất. Retrieved July 17, 2019, from http://khicongydaododucngoc.blogspot.com

203.Ngoc D. Duc. (n.d.). Ý nghĩa và công dụng chữa bệnh của những bài tập khí công, và giải đáp thắc mắc. 2015. Retrieved July 17, 2019, from http://khicongydaododucngoc.blogspot.com

204.O'Brien E (January 2001). Blood pressure measurement is changing!. Heart. 85 (1): 3–5. doi:10.1136/heart.85.1.3. PMC 1729570. PMID 11119446.

205.Ogedegbe G, Pickering T (November 2010). Principles and techniques of blood pressure measurement. Cardiology Clinics. 28 (4): 571–86.

206.Pankova A, Kralikova E, Zvolska K, et al Early weight gain after stopping smoking: a predictor of overall large weight gain? A single-site retrospective cohort study BMJ Open 2018;8:e023987. doi: 10.1136/bmjopen-2018-023987

207.Post RE, Dickerson LM (August 2010). Dizziness: a diagnostic approach. Am Fam Physician. 82 (4): 361–8, 369. PMID 20704166.

208.Reeves, Alexander G.; Swenson, Rand S. (2008). Chapter 14: Evaluation of the Dizzy Patient. Disorders of the Nervous System: A Primer. Dartmouth Medical School.

209.Remarkable recovery of seven-year-old girl. Jan 17, 2011. Archived from the original on 7 March 2015. Retrieved 2 March 2015.

210.Robertson, David (2012). Primer on the autonomic nervous system (3rd ed.). Amsterdam: Elsevier/AP. p. 288. ISBN 9780123865250. Archived from the original on 2017-09-08.

211.Van D. Dao. (September, 2017). AWAKEN YOU WONDERFUL WE: The secret of one-page table reveal all the real causes of all phenomena and problems:Most phenomena, physical problems, mental problems, social problems and how to solve them: Ability, Autoimmune diseases, Belief system, Gut feelings, Hysteria, Learning, Learning difficulties, Mental problems, ADHD, Alcohol use disorders, Anxiety disorders, Autism, Behavioral disorders, Depression,... https://www.amazon.com/Awaken-you-wonderful-phenomena-problems/dp/1549843524

212.What Is Hypothermia? Archived 2014-01-16 at the Wayback Machine

213.Worldwide trends in blood pressure from 1975 to 2015: a pooled analysis of 1479 population-based measurement studies with 19•1 million participants. The Lancet. 389 (10064): 37–55. January 2017.

Table of Contents

We will discuss in this book how to self-removing the trigger point and balancing metabolic reactions 2

This book is dedicated to 5

Chapter I: New view of self healing.....................................1

1.   In practice as a pharmacist, I found new view of pain, diseases and self healing. 1

Table 1: Self-checking the health and trigger points before, during and after practicing self-healing techniques or any other treatment..3

Table 2: Self-healing techniques and physical therapies that boost blood circulation, ...4

Physiotherapy can help but too complicated for all..................8

The health symptoms and diseases can benefit from these exercises: 8

Table 3: Mechanism of alternative therapies that help to prevent and heal chronic illness aim at nutritions and removing harmful wastes and clearing the vessels 10

Table 4: Top ten causes of death in high income/affluent countries – lifestyle diseases 12

2. Effect of deep breathing, Vietnamese Qi Gong exercise, and smoking on glycemia. 14

Table 5: Effect of different breathing on the blood pressure, glycemia and metabolism of the body....................................16

Chapter II: The relation between smoking, breathing, glycemia and the rate of the metabolism that reveals the effective way of controlling body weight and glycemia. 21

3. Body weight, smoking, feeling of hunger and glycemia 21

Table 6: Variations of diastolic pressure during practice these techniques..23

135

4. Effect of breathings on the glycemia in Khi Cong Y Dao Vietnam. 25

Chapter III. Self-removing the trigger points in the lungs to treat COVID-19, Corona, flu, flu A, cough, asthma, bronchitis, pneumonitis, and COPD..28

5. Practical view for self-finding and self-removing the trigger points in the lungs to treat COVID-19, Corona, flu, flu A, cough, asthma, bronchitis, pneumonitis, COPD, chest pain, coughing, difficulty breathing, tonsillitis, rhinitis. 28

Quickly and slightly punch on the back or on the chest under which there are the lungs, if there are places that the patients feel hurt, pain, breathlessness, causing the coughing or feel comfortable these are the trigger points that can make the lungs ill or pneumonitis. The trigger points I usually find are on the bottom of the lungs. We can remove these trigger points in the lungs by continuous punching on the lungs and the bottom of the lungs, which are the site of trigger points, for about 10 minutes each time. By asking the feeling of the patients and the sound during punching on the back we can know whether or not the trigger points have been removed? 28

You may feel like this is similar to postural drainage. No, this is better. The postural drainage technique makes patients feel lots of roughness on the back but does not make the lungs vibrate much. Punching on the back makes the whole lungs vibrate, this will make patients breathe easier. Do this in the right degree can be seen as a massage for the lungs to boost the health of the lungs. To know how much the vibration of the vessels and cells in the lungs, just quickly punching on the table, and see the vibrations of dust and objects on the table. If we can punch with a quick rhythm, we can make the lungs vibrate most with the little effort. The more we do for patients, the better the patients feel..28

Cough is the body reflex when having some problems or stuck in the airway...29

Epidemiology of COVID-19, the view that we may forget......29

6.   Steps to help treat flu, flu A, COVID-19, cold, difficult breathing, coughing, asthma, bronchitis, COPD, pneumonitis, chest pain and flu complications. 33

These steps together can help to boost the lungs and other illnesses so that the respiratory diseases recovered faster and do not create any complications 33

A. Eat and drink first to warm up the body 33

B. Lie down and place an object on the lower abdomen, this will make the blood circulate well to the whole body 33

C. Removing the trigger points in the lungs..........................34

1.   Quickly and slightly punch on the back or on the chest under which there are the lungs, if there are places that the patients feel hurt, pain, breathlessness, trigger coughing or feel comfortable these are the trigger points that can make the lungs ill or pneumonitis. The trigger points I usually find are on the bottom of the lungs. We can remove these trigger points in the lungs by continuous punching on the lungs and the bottom of the lungs, which are the site of trigger points, for about 10 minutes each time. By asking the feeling of the patients and the sound during punching on the back we can know whether or not the trigger points have been removed? 34

2.   Continous doing these several days can remove all the forgotten trigger points in the lungs. After trigger points removed, clapping on the back just creates the normal feeling, no more the feeling hurt, pain, breathlessness or trigger coughing..34

D. Clapping on trigger points on the whole body until having the sensation of roughness..34

Aims that therapies should aim 35

Chapter IV. Keep the vessels at the optimum osmotic permeability 36

7. The vital role of circulation: 36

A. The functions of the blood 36

The blood platelets...37

The red blood cells 38

The white blood cells 38

B. The quality of blood can be found in blood test, in simple, practitioners can see the quality of blood by checking glycemia and blood pressure 38

C. The complication of diabetes may be explained that the cells are hungry for so long. 41

D. In a body, all in one, one in all. 42

E. The health of central nervous system 43

F. The constriction of the muscle cells, the narrowed vessels 44

8. Forget biology, forget the immune system when there are problems that reduce blood circulation. 47

Table 7: The signs and the effects of hypotension. 50

Changing lifestyle, adequate diet is the advice for most diseases 51

Chapter V. The vessels are the basic structures of the whole body. .54

9. There are four main types of blood vessels that each play their own role: 54

Table 8: There are four main types of blood vessels that each play their own role: 54

Structure of the blood vessels...55

10. Hormones and acts of medication on vessels..................57

Table 9: Side effects of three stress chemicals 58

Serious side effects cortisol...58

11. Forget medicines, forget modern techniques if cutting the
energy source for the cells..61

   A. Cells with metabolic reactions are the basic structure of all
tissues and organs...61

   Table 10: Catabolic reactions 61

   Table 11: The factors that impact the catabolic reactions in the
body...61

   B. Hypoglycemia and hypothermia..................................62

   Table 12: The signs and the effects of hypoglycemia 63

   C. Hypothermia 65

   Table 13: The signs and the effects of hypothermia..............65

12. Let the body to remove trigger point and balance metabolic
reactions 68

   Picture 1: Applications of the healingChapter VI: Self-healing
chronic diseases..72

13. Removing the trigger point and balancing metabolic reactions
are the keys to fatigue, backache, headache, leg pain,
neurodegenerative diseases, asthma, COPD, flu, fever, flu A, and
COVID-19...73

   A. Eat and drink first..74

   B. Lie down and place an object on the lower abdomen........75

   C. Relaxed deep breathing 76

   D. Clapping on the body to remove the trigger points until
having the sensation of roughness. 77

   E. Finding and removing trigger points in the lungs by
comfortable clapping or punching....................................77

   •   Quickly and slightly punch on the back or on the chest
under which there are the lungs, if there are places that the

patients feel hurt, pain, breathlessness, trigger coughing or feel comfortable these are the trigger points that can make the lungs ill or pneumonitis. The trigger points I usually find are on the bottom of the lungs. We can remove these trigger points in the lungs by continuous punching on the lungs and the bottom of the lungs, which are the site of trigger points, for about 10 minutes each time. By asking the feeling of the patients and the sound during punching on the back we can know whether or not the trigger points have been removed? 78

• Continous doing these several days can remove all the forgotten trigger points in the lungs. After trigger points removed, clapping on the back just creates the normal feeling, no more the feeling hurt, pain, breathlessness or trigger coughing. 78

F. Removing trigger points in the stomach by pulling the knee to the chest and blow the air deeply and slowly 78

G.   For varicose veins 79

H. For Insomnia 79

I. For eyes problems: 79

J. For hemorrhoid and constipation 79

K. Loading energy, boosting blood circulation for five important organs... 80

This exercise also used to test the health of the muscles of the legs, knees, and hips. If the blood circulation is not well, the practitioners may not stand in 2 minutes. 80

L. Boost the blood circulation and soften all muscles in hand, neck and shouder. 80

M. For nausea and vomitting.. 81

14.   Self-healing chronic diseases. 82

A.   Science of the Qi 82

Table 14: Balancing Qi 82

B.   All of the steps in this chapter can use to help healing many chronic diseases. 84

•   Warming the hand and feet and the whole body to reduce irritation, treat Raynaud, numbness and tingling in hands and feet, cold hands, feet, weakness and hands and legs 84

•   Irritation bowel, irritation on the stomach, gastric, flatulent, dyspepsia indigestion, or pain in the liver, hepatitis, prolonged diarrhea, or vomiting. 84

•   Insomnia, headache, dizziness, vertigo, floating, Alzheimer's, chronic fatigue and neurodegenerative Diseases, and Seizures 84

•   Hepatitis, liver inflammation, pancreatitis, jaundice, chronic itching, eczema, constipation, and irritation bowel movement, chronic diarrheas, menstrual pain, Dysuria (painful urination), and cramp. 84

•   Treating Sinusitis, rhinitis, blocking nose, faceache seasonal allergy, chronic coughing, pneumonia, poor sleeping, tuberculosis, and chronic respiratory problems......................85

•   Backache, neck pain, headache, shoulder pain, stiff neck, back pain, lumbar pain and nerve pain, numbness and tingling in hands and feet, cold hands, feet; the weakness...................85

Chapter VI: The cause and possible cure metabolic disorders and cancers. 86

15.   The cause and possible cure metabolic disorders and cancers.86

A. Possible results of metabolic disorders prove that metabolic disorders are the real cause...87

B. Oxidative stress 87

C. Neuritis is the general inflammation of the peripheral nervous system that may link to Parkinson's diseases, Leprosy, and diabetic complications. 88

D. Carcinogen 88

E. Pain in many illnesses and in fibromyalgia 89

F. Other medical conditions that share similar symptoms as systemic metabolic disorders that need to have deeper research. .89

Chapter VII: The mind: stress and inner peace. 92

16.   The brain with obsessed desires 92

    A.   Human needs explaining by Abraham Maslow: 93

    B.   Human needs explained by Tony Robbins....................93

    What do the human needs mean?..94

17. STRESS MEANS PROBLEMS ARE BIGGER THAN ABILITIES..96

    Table 12: Effects of three stress chemicals 98

    Serious side effects cortisol..98

    READ FIGHT, FLIGHT or INDIFFERENCE SIGNALS.....99

18. The role of meditation to have a healthy, happy life 101

    Picture 2: sitting postures of meditation...............................102

    A. Buddhism meditation..103

    B. Simple mediation practices for busy people:....................107

    Exercise one: Observe the relaxation of the whole body.....108

    Exercise two: Observe the breath. 108

    Exercise three: Count the breath during meditating 108

    Exercise four: observe the lower abdomen............................108

    Exercise five: Observe the lower body in meditating...........109

Exercise six: identify the thoughts that appear from the top of the head 110

C. Mindfulness prevents us from making mistakes..............112

D. People may be lead to crazy emotion if they lack mindfulness 115

E. Mindful reading to emotional management 117

ALL IN ONE, ONE IN ALL: 118

References: 119

Table of Contents 139

www.ingramcontent.com/pod-product-compliance
Lightning Source LLC
Chambersburg PA
CBHW030648220526
45463CB00005B/1680